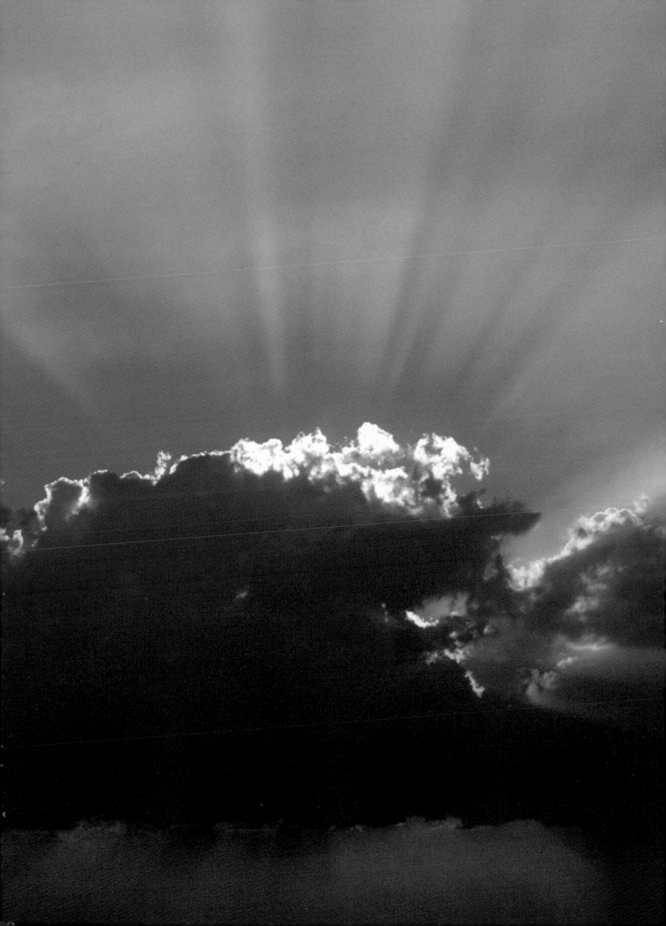

Library of Congress

Deja Vu Lifestyle Creations, LLC
7657 Berkshire Pines Drive
Suite 1609
Naples, FL 34104
Orders: www.evolvewithflavor.com

Design by Amy Fisher, Fisher Graphics, Inc.

Cover photo by Gary Jung/**garyjung**.com

Photographs of Rabbit Run Farm courtesy of Denise Muir, Owner

ISBN: 978-0-9836531-0-3

Printed in China

For our families,

with special places in each of our hearts

for Opa and Grampy.

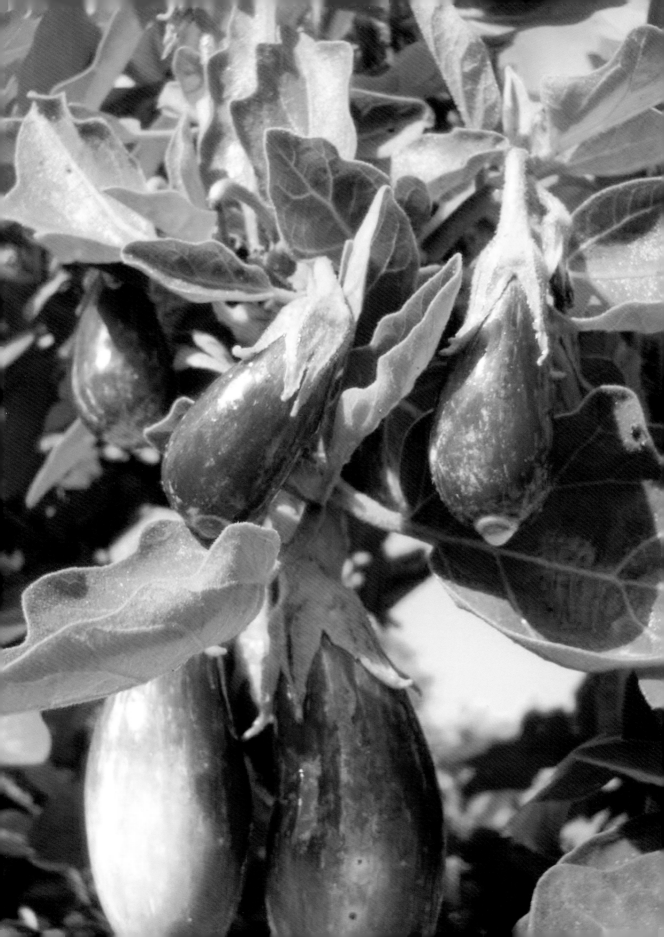

Acknowledgements

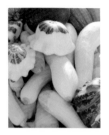

My sincerest thank you...

To my beautiful wife, Judy. My most special thanks go to her, for without her time-consuming efforts, this book would never have become a reality. Not only is she creative and ultra intelligent, she also has the capacity to grasp how I want my recipes to read and my thoughts expressed. She was the artistic force behind this book–from the overall design, to the photographic elements to the prose. I thank her for all of that and for her love and patience.

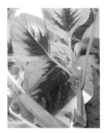

To Debra van Schaardenberg for being my nutritional sherpa, my guide through the world of healthy blood and the foods that help get it that way. Not only did she unselfishly open her home to me and all of the class attendees, while pulling the classes together administratively, she spear-headed the whole idea of doing the classes in the first place.

To Denise Muir and her Rabbit Run Farm, where her hydroponically grown organic vegetables and fruits are some of the most beautiful and delicious this side of Eden. Her produce is an inspiration.

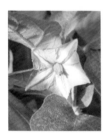

To Amy Fisher of Fisher Graphics... for her creative professionalism, her witty, infectious sense of humor, and for bringing our dream to life.

To all of my friends, family and class attendees who encouraged me to persevere and "write that book".

A warm thank you from Judy...

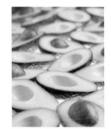

To my sister, Lyn Breedon, for her unconditional love and support and for being my sounding board. Whatever did I do without her for the first two and a half years of my life?

To Eileen Wesley for being a rock and a shoulder at the same time.

To Dr. Molly Barrow for helping me to see through it all.

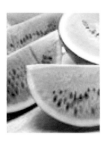

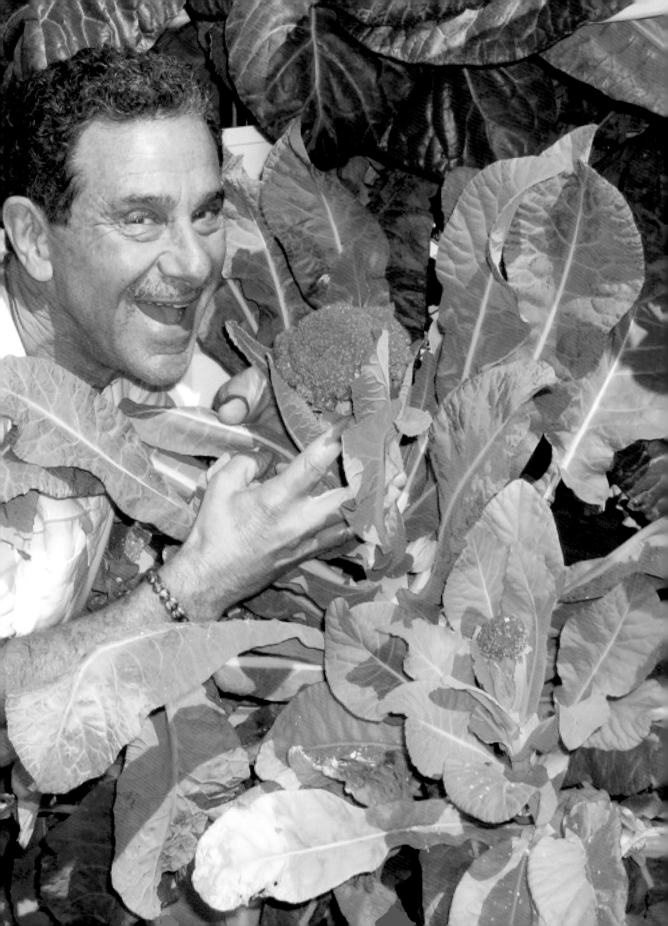

Table of Contents

DISCOVERING

RAW
ALKALINE

CUISINE

Through Love, Passion and Health

One Chef's Journey

Recipes

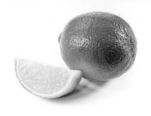

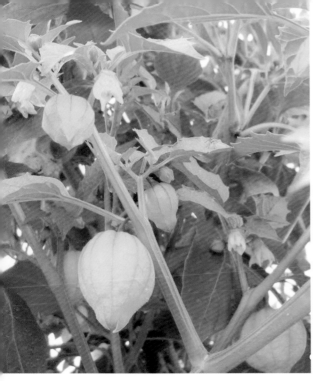

DIPS, ETC.

DRESSINGS

SALADS

SAUCES

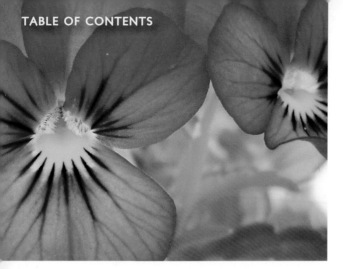

MEAL MENU SUGGESTIONS

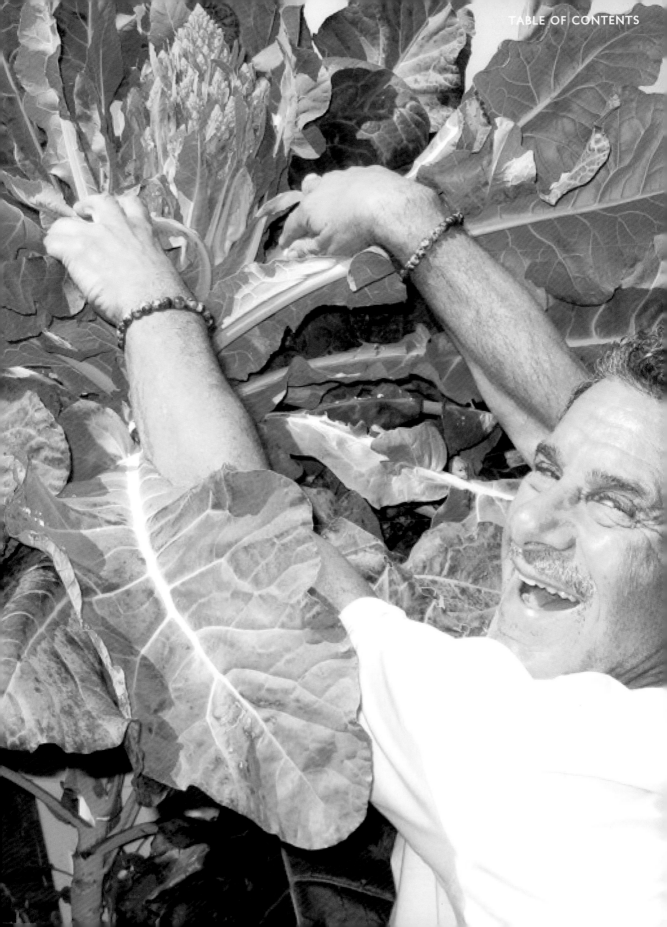

Introduction

An Introduction to Easy, Delicious Raw Alkaline Cuisine
Through Love, Passion and Health

Exactly who am I, and what's in this book for you?

I am a chef. It is my passion…it is what I love. I am not a doctor, a dietician, a nutritionist, or a scientist. I am a human being that has experienced the results on my body of a variety of different foods and diets over my lifetime. Through the different phases of my life, I have come to appreciate the feeling of extreme well being when I ingest a diet of raw, alkaline forming foods. I combine my diet regimen with an exercise routine that works best for me; I am happy to be in this space and time.

The mere fact that you have even picked up this book indicates that you must have at least an interest in increasing the quality of your life through your food choices. You may even already be an advocate for a raw diet, an alkaline diet, or a combination of both. There are millions of words that you can find today in bookstores and on the internet that will help guide you in your own journey to achieving your best through proper sustenance.

This book is not intended to indoctrinate you into the life of a raw, alkaline diet per se. This book is my answer to the often-asked question: "where can I find raw, alkaline recipes for meals that taste good?" No one seems to have come up with the answer. Using my many years of experience as an award winning chef, I sought to try to find the improbable mix of healthy, yet delicious raw cuisine. I believe that I have indeed succeeded, and I know that those that have eaten this food agree.

Life is all about love, passion and health…we strive to attain the best of these. I am blessed to have an abundance of all three: my family and friends, my cooking and never-ending enthusiasm for that delicious yet healthy dish, along with my increased robust feelings of vitality, athleticism and just plain agelessness.

The love and passion in my life have been with me in many ways. The love that survived long after loved ones have gone, the love that continues to grow with all those that are here, and the love of friends that I am sure I am yet to meet.

The passion I attained by building each of my restaurants into fine dining establishments and creating award-winning meals for my guests to enjoy has fueled me for over 50 years.

The health part of my life has been a longer learning journey. I believed that I was blessed with near-perfect health; over the years I discovered I was not. I was born in 1938 and through the many experiences of my life—from the acutely painful to the most exhilarating times of joy — I found myself on the verge of a new experience. I began this chapter of my life in Naples, Florida, in 2004. This is where my journey to extreme health and revitalized youth really came home to me; some wonderful people were put in my path that reached out to help me and shared the knowledge they gained through their life's experiences. I realized that I had to make some changes to achieve that near-perfect health that I thought I sought. I took the gifts of knowledge I received from my friends and incorporated them into my own daily regimen.

I have found a new, healthy awakening in myself; I am revitalized; I feel younger than I did many years ago. My understanding of — and partaking in — raw alkaline fitness foods has provided me with the insight to draw on my 50 years of creating fine dining cuisine into conceiving the most delicious raw, alkaline based meals through which everyone may enjoy and prosper. Now I am reaching out to help you…with wishes for the best of life, through love, passion and health.

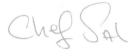

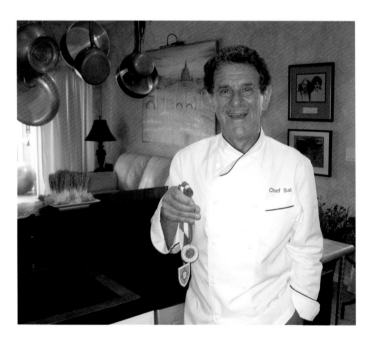

My Journey

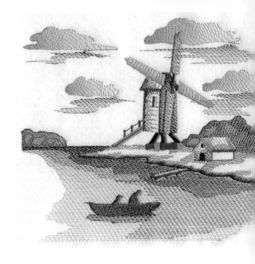

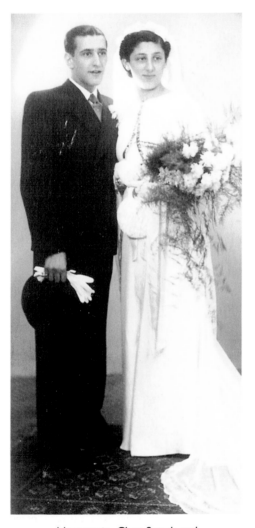

My parents, Clara Swaab and
Raphaël Montezinos on their wedding day
in Amsterdam.

I was born in Amsterdam, Holland, The Netherlands on June 22, 1938, the first child of very young, hard-working, successful and loving parents. My family is of Jewish descent, the first Montezinos arrived in The Netherlands from Portugal in the 1500s. My mother's family owned a renowned cigar store in Amsterdam's center; she cared for me at home while my father honed his skills as a designer and tailor for the actors and actresses at the nearby Carré Theater. We lived across the canal; I watched the actors and actresses come and go into the theater from my window. We had a wonderful, happy life – that was to end soon.

November 9 through 10, 1938 Kristallnacht (The Night of Broken Glass) terrorized Jews throughout Europe in Nazi-controlled areas. Not long after that, my parents were rounded up, taken by train to the concentration camp in Westerbork, The Netherlands. This was a detention and transit camp; its function was to assemble the Romani people and Dutch Jews for transport to other Nazi concentration camps. My parents were in fact transported to Dachau, where they were annihilated.

The day that my parents were picked up, my grandfather overheard some Nazi soldiers talking about their day's activities and the areas in which Jews would be picked up for transport. My grandfather knew where I was playing street soccer and swooped in, picked me up and hid me for a time. He finally found a Christian family that lived on a farm on the outskirts of Amsterdam; they took me to live with them, gave me a Christian name, and brought me to church with them on Sundays. I was so young and not completely aware of what was happening at the time I spent at the farm.

I experienced some awful sights along with some wonderful feelings of the senses. I spent a good deal of the war hiding in the barn on the farm; sometimes I would hear terrible noises, look out the barn's open windows and see airplanes falling to the ground with plumes of smoke coming from them. I was so scared, so lonely to be by myself, hiding in that barn. Yet, other times I was happy being at the farm, playing with the animals and partaking in some of the best, freshest vegetables and fruits. Even now, when I eat a particularly delicious piece of organic fruit, it brings me immediately back to being that little boy…the reliving of the enjoyment of the taste of that food is one of only a few sustaining happy memories from that time. After the liberation, I was sent to an orphanage for Jewish children, just outside the Amsterdam city limits. I lived there, was schooled there, and in my teens went out the windows at night to go to jazz clubs with my friends in the city. After a year or so after arriving at the orphanage, the headmaster called me into his office; he then brought in a little girl, whom he introduced to me as my sister Elly. I had no idea I even had a sister – she was only a few months old when my parents were picked up, but I was too young for any memory of her. Elly lives in Amsterdam today, surrounded by her friends and the remainder of our family.

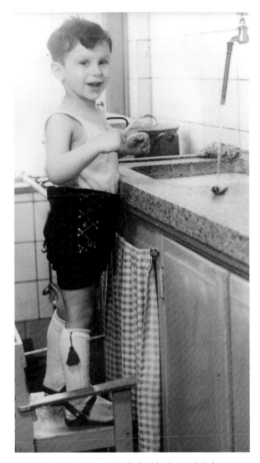

Age 4 at our family's kitchen sink in Amsterdam. A sign of things to come perhaps?

When I was old enough to leave the orphanage at age 17, I got involved in the hospitality industry, first with a part ownership in a small "Sundays Only" jazz spot in Hilversum, then moving on to hotel school and working in some of Amsterdam's finest restaurants. At a very young age, I met a beautiful girl, and we married. I was happy; we moved to Switzerland, where my son Edward came along, and I knew just how happy I could be. The mother of my beautiful young wife, however, did not see me as a success at the time, believing her daughter could do better. She banished me from the house, wielding a butcher knife. It was heartbreaking for me, particularly to leave Edward. He is now a very smart, successful man, living near Amsterdam, with two sons of his own. After I was forced to leave, I was lost. I continued my culinary studies in The Netherlands for a while; but I had wanderlust. I wanted to see, smell and taste other places, foreign shores, all the while moving forward with my calling.

I travelled, studied and trained in the culinary and hospitality arts in Switzerland, France, Singapore, Israel and Spain. It was while working on European cruise lines as a dining room captain that I made the decision to go to the United States and open a restaurant.

In 1970 I arrived in Philadelphia, Pennsylvania. At the time, I spoke five languages, but English was a very, very foreign language to me. In what seemed to be just a blur of time, I became versed in English, met and married the most beautiful woman in the world, rented a space in an

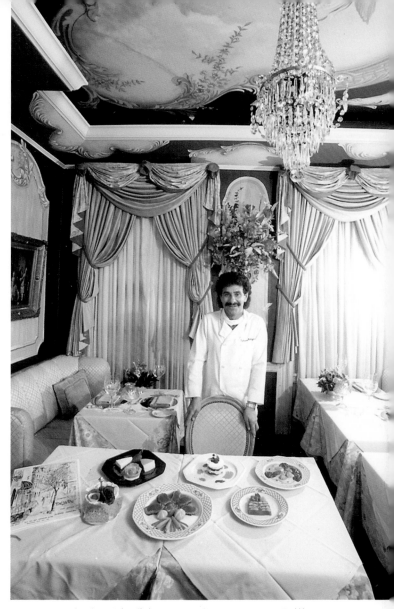

In the main dining room of my restaurant, Déjà vu, in Philadelphia, Pennsylvania.

1800s brick townhouse in downtown Philadelphia and turned it into a casual café. In time I bought the entire townhouse, renovated it and lived with my wife, Susan, on the top floors, and turned the bottom floors into one of the grandest, award-winning restaurants in the United States…Déjà vu. The restaurant was gorgeous; it was written up in all of the most prestigious gourmet magazines. One writer proclaimed, "10 Tables; 5,000 Bottles of Wine!" Life was exciting; it couldn't get any better; then in April 1975 it did. Our daughter Danielle was born.

The three of us lived happy lives for many years in the old Philadelphia brownstone that housed both our home and Déjà vu. I cooked, oversaw the staff and ran the day-to-day function of the restaurant. Susan took care of our home and our daughter. The restaurant was the focus of our world. So much so that one night Francis Ford Coppola came in for dinner and offered me a bit part in his latest upcoming movie, The Godfather III, but I turned it down, telling him "I am too busy." I can laugh now, but that's a tough memory to digest. However, I do still have the page he signed in the guest book that night, declaring Déjà vu "The Finest Restaurant in the World!!" Framed of course. Although I hosted many celebrities in my restaurants over the years, I keep Francis Coppola's signature as a reminder of a lesson well learned. Don't be too busy to look up once in a while; if you don't, you just might let something really special slip away.

After nearly fifteen years of growing, nurturing and living Déjà vu, Susan and I started to get restless. In the mid-1980s we sold the house, and along with the restaurant, packed up and moved to Palm Beach, Florida. For the next twelve years, I had the pleasure of opening and running three successful culinary establishments, two eponymous restaurants, Montezinos, in Orlando and Palm Beach, and the lovely Angelique in Boca Raton. It was in these restaurants that I expand-

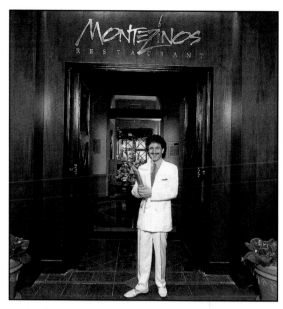

At the entrance to Montezinos Restaurant in Orlando, Florida.

ed and refocused my repertoire of menu items to concentrate on the seafood and organic fresh fruits and vegetables that are abundant in the tropical environment that exist in The Sunshine State. I loved working with the products that came directly to me from the ocean and the local organic farms. The aroma and flavor of those fruits, vegetables and seafood brought back the few happy memories I had of being hidden on that small farm outside of Amsterdam during the war. Just smelling and eating those foods gave me a feeling of happiness.

I loved the experience of learning more about the healthy aspects of certain foods, honing my skills and still being able to bring smiles to the faces of my customers by presenting them with delicious fare. I put all I had into my three restaurants, all of me; I literally had no time for anything else. As any chef that has owned and operated a restaurant will tell you, your life is not your own—the restaurant consumes you 24 hours a day — and I had three. My agenda was crazy, and naturally my schedule affected my wife and daughter. They wanted to spend more time together as a family, and quite frankly, I was beginning to tire of hurtling up and down I-95 from Orlando to Palm Beach and Boca Raton — very often in blinding Florida rainstorms.

After much soul searching, I decided to give up my existence as a hands-on owner/chef/restaurateur. At least for a while. I made a huge change in my life by trying on a career as executive chef in a number of well-known restaurants in south Florida. I continued to work with and learn the ins and outs of organic produce and fresh-caught bounty from the ocean. Still, being a chef — even an executive chef — for someone else on a daily basis was not something that made me feel whole. My family and I were happy to have more time together, but I felt unfulfilled in my having to march to someone else's drum. For the most part, the menus and recipes were long

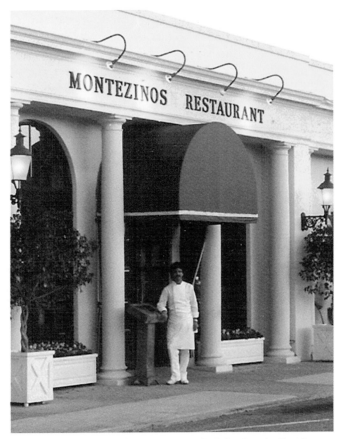

Outside of Montezinos Restaurant in Palm Beach, Florida.

established in these restaurants; my passion fell a few notches.

I was then presented with a wonderful opportunity to become the corporate executive chef for a small group of restaurants…there were three at the time, located in Florida, Chicago and Hawaii. Within this capacity I was able to develop menus and recipes, train the staff on achieving the perfect preparation of each dish, and in essence oversee and run the kitchens. I was much happier, much more fulfilled with my career. Believe it or not, even though I was flying from Florida to Chicago to Hawaii and back often, I was actually spending more time with my family than I was during the years I owned my three restaurants in Florida.

Of course, not so deep down, I did miss having my own restaurants, creating all of the dishes and being my own boss. I did not, however, regret my decision to walk away from my restaurants to be surrounded with the joy and happiness that my family provided. I had the realization, as do so many others, that some things are just meant to be. They may be attached to disappointment and some level of malcontent, and it may take years to understand just why things worked out the way they did, but one usually figures it out. Looking back, I could not have made a better judgment those years before than to place my restaurant dreams on a shelf and to put my family first.

Danielle had since gone off to college in New York, and Susan and I were living the empty-nest syndrome in Florida. Susan began to mention that she was not feeling completely well, and that she missed her family and friends in Philadelphia – not to mention that we were so far away from New York and Danielle. It is ironic that at a time when I was starting to feel healthier than ever that Susan was feeling listless, out of sorts and just not one hundred percent.

Coincidentally, the small group of restaurants for which I worked as corporate executive chef in Florida, Chicago and Hawaii was opening a fourth restaurant – a very upscale, fine dining

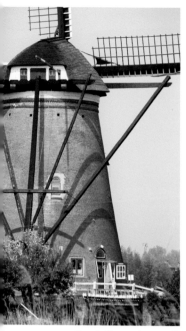

establishment in a first-class hotel/condominium on Rittenhouse Square in Philadelphia. I was offered a position there as executive chef, whereby I would have control over the kitchen staff as well as the opportunity to develop menus and recipes. Susan and I decided to make our way back to Philadelphia...to our extensive family and friends, to my regaining a strong passion for my occupation and to continue working on a healthy, anti-aging regimen for us both.

Our lives were moving along nicely in Philadelphia; and because we were close to New York, we were able to see Danielle fairly often. Susan was feeling good again; we thought that perhaps her ill feelings in Florida were partly tied up in homesickness. I was enjoying my career and new station in life. In fact, we had really settled in; everything seemed to be going as we had hoped and anticipated.

Then the unthinkable happened. Susan's feelings of ill health returned, but this time with a vengeance. She was diagnosed with pancreatic cancer and told that she had about three months to live. On Sunday, May 14, 2000 – Mother's Day – surrounded by her family, her best friend, Danielle and myself, Susan left us. Yet she is still with us every day.

I was devastated. However, I knew then with the utmost clarity that I had made the right decision in Florida to give up my restaurants in order to focus on the people I loved the most in this world. There was a reason. I also knew that I had no idea how to get beyond the grief and sadness that I woke up with and went to bed with every single day.

One of the things Susan instilled in me was to have the courage to go after my dreams, always encouraging me, telling me I could achieve anything that I wanted. I kept those positive thoughts next to my heart and tried to live by them on a day-to-day basis. Through this process I met some wonderful new friends and opened myself up to embracing a spirituality that I had previously only brushed by. My work had left little time for reflection and meditation; now I felt an overwhelming need for just that. So I threw myself into getting to know myself again. I reflected on my life up to that point and meditated on more ethereal ideals. I began exercising, running, working out at the gym, eating a healthy diet, learning about the effects of foods, minerals, enzymes, vitamins and positive thoughts on the body.

Danielle and I took a trip to visit my family in The Netherlands to reconnect. I had seen them all from time to time through the years and was happy to spend some time with them again. My sister, my aunts, uncles and cousins. My son, Edward had married and would have a son of his own within the year. I made a promise to move forward, get healthy, live within the love that Susan left behind for me, and get my passion back. It took a lot of fortitude that I wasn't sure I had. But I was beginning to heal.

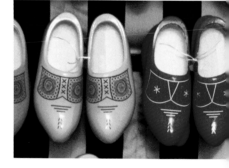

A year passed. I had made it through with the help of my friends and family. It was a very difficult time for me; Susan was gone after 30 years together. Luckily we had an energetic, bright, talented daughter; just knowing she was here was a particularly great comfort to me.

I had a lot of time on my hands. I took that time get to know myself better, to more deeply explore my spirituality, my inner strength, my thirst for knowledge in all aspects of my life. I perfected my meditation methods and started taking yoga instructions, which developed into my participation in regularly-scheduled classes. My exercise program became more of a practiced rhythm through yoga, running for the aerobic benefits and weight training.

I also spent a lot of time investigating and analyzing different ways of cooking, beyond my years of gourmet expertise. Years before, I had discovered ways that I could create delicious sauces — without adding a drop of cream or a pat of butter — by reducing fresh organic herbs, fruits and vegetables while adding a few extra flourishes.

I decided to work with those principal foundations and expand them into different food group areas that would promote a healthier course of eating. I tested the waters of the outside world by consulting and developing dishes for a number of health-food-conscious cafes. I was finally on my way again, with a renewed spirit and determination, along with an unchartered horizon in view.

Fate, once again, set its sights on changing my life. One stupendously bright Sunday morning in the spring of 2001, I was standing on the edge of Rittenhouse Square, talking to a friend. It was one of those magnificent days that Mother Nature trots out from to time; the sky was totally blue, without a cloud, and just a hint of a chill in the air. I spotted a woman walking in my direction. She had something — I couldn't quite see what it was — sticking out of her jacket. The "something" the woman had sticking out of her jacket turned out to be the cutest cat I had ever seen, her oh-so fluffy Himalayan cat, Perri. The woman's name was Judy Castille. We were married a year and a half later on the Caribbean island of Grenada.

In December 2004 Judy and I moved to Naples, Florida. Judy's sister and brother-in-law, Lyn and George, had moved to Naples late in 1987 and fell in love with it. When they decided to move, they just left their jobs, packed up their life and made that huge leap. They are successful and happy here today.

We were encouraged by their enterprising actions and thought that a move to Florida ourselves would be great. Judy had been to Naples to visit a number of times over the years, and of course I had lived in a number of cities on the other coast of Florida; we enjoyed it here. So, we too packed up our life and moved to Naples.

During our first year in Naples, I did a lot of personal chef work, catering and consulting. Through this work I met a number of people with diverse backgrounds and lives, along with a significant appreciation for a healthy body, attitude and longevity. I had the pleasure of learning something from each of these people and through them was able to expand my depth of knowledge in a variety of areas. I was becoming more and more interested in raw cuisine and was testing out recipes.

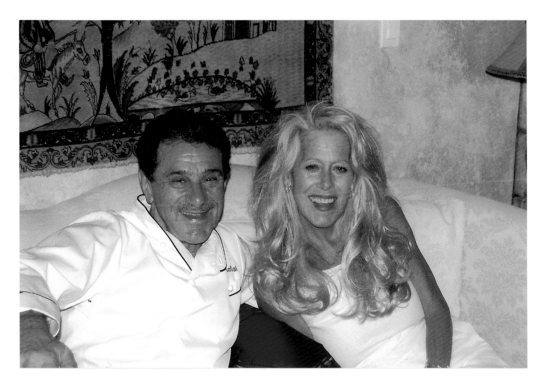

At home with my wife, Judy, in Naples, Florida.

At that time I met a very interesting woman named Debra Van Schaardenberg who is extremely knowledgeable about the effects of certain diets and how one's blood reacts to those foods. During the course of the time I spent developing healthy, raw, alkaline-based recipes, I would discuss these dishes with Debra. We both agreed that my recipes could help in alleviating certain detrimental blood issues.

At that point people were asking me to give classes on how to make delicious raw food cuisine and requesting copies of the recipes. It was Debra that had the spark of an idea to put the recipes into some sort of book form. She also gave me a great gift in opening her own home in which to hold the classes. In fact, she oversaw the details regarding the attendance of the classes; she made phone calls, sent e-mails, and brought in new class members.

My journey thus far has brought me here. I set out to produce a book with delicious recipes that are not easy to find in the world of raw cuisine. Through this book I also want to share the things I do to keep the love, passion and health in my life. Many angels have been placed in my way to get me to this point; perhaps through this book I can be one for you.

The Scoop on Alkaline-Based Food

I recommend eating an 80-20% alkaline to acid based diet.
So why did I write a book filled with 100% alkaline-based
recipes? Here's the deal. I give you recipes to make the most
of the 80% raw alkaline portion of your diet regimen;
you decide on the remaining 20%.

Remember that whatever you choose to eat, always treat your body with respect. Do not treat it like a garbage receptacle. You will be healthier and happier for it.

If you have done any research on alkaline and acidic diets, I am sure that you have come across hundreds of references. There are arguments for all-alkaline diets, arguments for all-acid diets and arguments for balanced alkaline-acid diets as well. Set within these hundreds of references are hundreds of opinions—just what foods are considered alkaline and which are considered acidic—it can get very confusing out there.

For the most part, however, there is a basic consensus on just what is what. A rule of thumb is that alkaline-based foods consist of fruits, vegetables, grains, nuts and seeds—while acid-based foods consist of foods rich in sugars, flours and saturated fats, such as meats, dairy products, pasta, bread, etc.

Many diets that you may be familiar with are either alkaline or acid based, but are not necessarily referred to that way. They have names like Atkins, Zone and Stillman and they focus on high protein/low carbohydrates, high carbohydrates/low fat and various combinations thereof. Most of these diets are followed by people in an effort to lose weight. Weight might be the least of what is lost by adhering to any all-or-nothing diet: important minerals and vitamins essential to our bodies are lost as well.

There is a consensus that a raw, alkaline-based diet can help you lose weight. Naturally, ceasing to eat foods that are high in sugar, flour, and fat only stands to reason that you most likely would lose weight. Using this diet *simply* to lose weight is not its purpose; however if you choose to eat this way to achieve a weight goal, you will also receive many other—perhaps unexpected—benefits.

It is important to understand how the combination of alkaline and acid forming foods work within our bodies to achieve and sustain normal pH levels. The foods we eat will leave behind either an alkaline or an acid ash once the food has been metabolized.

That ash has a direct effect on the pH levels in your body. pH refers to the *power of Hydrogen*, meaning the concentration of hydrogen ions present in a substance. The neutral pH level is 7; water for instance has a pH level of 7. The pH levels in foods above 7 are alkaline forming foods; conversely, the pH levels in foods below 7 are acid forming. You can test your own pH level easily with an over-the-counter pH strip kit; these strips can be swabbed with your saliva or held in your urine stream. Your doctor can test your pH through your blood with an easy test.

The normal pH level for blood is 7.41; for urine, it falls in a range of between 4.5 to 8. If the pH level in our bodies falls out of range, our bodies will try to correct it, but the pH level can be helped with the correct diet. A pH level that is too high or too low is not where we want to be. If there is too much alkaline ash in our bodies, bringing our pH levels too high, it can result in alkalosis, while too much acid ash can result in a very low pH, bringing on acidosis.

Both of these conditions have their own negative symptoms and side effects. However, parasites, mold, yeast and generally bad bacteria cannot exist in an alkaline environment while dietary phosphates exist in acid environments which bind to calcium and prevent our bodies from absorbing it.

It is my belief that a balanced alkaline-acid diet works best for us. In "balanced", I am not referring to a 50-50% mix. Instead, I believe that an 80-20% ratio of alkaline to acid foods is the foremost mix for our bodies in regard to health, well being and age-hindering aspects.

You will note that the title of my book is in part *Discovering Raw Alkaline Cuisine*, and that it is a book filled with 100% alkaline-only-based recipes. That fact seems to be at odds with the argument for an 80-20% ratio diet. After all, I'm providing recipes that are 100% alkaline—where's that 80-20 breakdown? Well, that's up to you. I'm giving you ways to make delicious foods for the 80% of your diet... you choose the remaining 20% to your liking.

For the purposes of this book, I have put together delicious raw dishes that are made with all alkaline-based foods. I am also providing you with lists of both alkaline-based as well as acid-based foods. There are a few foods that are not on these lists that you may find on other alkaline-based approved food lists; I believe that the lists I have put together work best. My advice to you is to follow the 80-20% rule; adhere to the 80% alkaline intake through the use of my recipes and add a limited amount of acid-based foods of your liking into your daily regimen. Of course that 80-20% ratio is my suggestion; that percentage could be modified to your liking. You will make the determination of the percentages based on how you feel. I decided to write this book and share my recipes for those of you looking for healthy, yet delicious, satisfying meals, working within a balance.

I was developing recipes for classes in—and teaching the art of—raw cooking when a number of my class attendees came to me with very specific and often serious health problems. I set out to investigate further the effects of diet and proper pH levels on the body to see if there was some additional way in which I could help these people.

At that time, I was deeply ensconced in the belief that raw cuisine was a healthy way to eat and found myself just naturally gravitating toward foods that I later learned were considered to be alkaline.

Although I was unintentionally already developing recipes with an alkaline focus, I discovered through my research that certain fruits and vegetables were not the best for our bodies. I found hundreds of cookbooks and websites geared toward raw cuisine. I also found quite a number of cookbooks and websites specifically for alkaline or acid forming foods.

However, I found a dearth of books and websites for recipes that fit the criteria that was most important to me: raw, easy to make, alkaline based, healthy, pH balanced, and delicious... all in one place. *Delicious* was of utmost importance to me... I wanted to taste, eat and serve food that looked and tasted like the cooked food it was replacing. What I found were a lot of recipes that had names like the foods most of us grew up eating, yet many were served in bowls and came in varying textures of oatmeal or gruel and in a boring variety of colors that spanned the gray and brown spectrums. That aspect of those foods has slowly started to come around.

So there it was; I saw a need. However, I also saw a pretty empty space when I went to find specific answers; I was on a mission. So I took my 50 plus years of experience, my need to help others and my desire to create delicious food and jumped right into that empty space.

As I said at the beginning of this book, I am not a doctor, a nutritionist or a scientist. I am, however, an acclaimed, healthy chef. I have developed delicious recipes for raw, alkaline-based meals that work for me, and I am passing them along to you. Please make sure that you check with your doctor or wellness care giver prior to changing your eating habits or beginning a diet of any kind.

Acid Forming Food Items

Alcoholic Beverages	Cereals	Egg Whites	Ice Cream	Pickled Olives	Spaghetti
Bananas, Green	Cheeses, All	Fish and Shellfish	Indian Teas	Plums	Sugar, Refined
Barley	Coloring, Artificial	Flavoring, Artificial	Jams and Jellies	Prunes	Tabasco
Beans, Dried	Condiments, All	Flour Products	Lentils	Rice, White and Brown	Tapioca
Breads	Corn, Cooked	Garbanzos	Mayonnaise	Salt, Regular Table	Vinegar, Other Than Apple Cider
Cakes	Corn Starch	Gelatin	Meats and Poultry	Soda Water	Yogurt
Candy	Crackers	Grains	Oatmeal	Soft Drinks	
Canned Fruits and Vegetables	Cranberries	Grapenuts	Pasta	Soy Beans	
	Custards	Gravies	Pastries and Pies	Soy Products	
	Dairy Products	Hominy Grits	Peanuts		
	Doughnuts				

Alkaline Forming Fruits

Apples	Milk	Guava	Melons, All	Pineapple
Apricots	Oil	Kumquats	Nectarines	Pomegranates
Bananas	Water	Lemons	Noni	Prickly Pear
Berries	Currants	Limes	Passion Fruit	Raisins
Cherries	Dates	Longanberries	Papaya	Sapotes
Coconut	Figs	Loquats	Pears	Strawberries
Butter	Grapefruit	Mangos	Peaches	Tamarind
Meat	Grapes			

Alkaline Forming Oils

Avocado Oil	Extra Virgin Olive Oil	Hemp Seed Oil	Safflower Oil
Black Current Oil	Flaxseed Oil	Pumpkin Seed Oil	Salba Oil
Coconut Oil	Grape Seed Oil	Red Palm Oil	Wheat Germ Oil

Alkaline Forming Miscellaneous Food Items

Agave	Herbal Teas	Millet	Quinoa	Hijiki
Amaranth	Himalayan Sea Salt	Miso	Sea Vegetables	Kelp
Apple Cider Vinegar	Horseradish	Nama Shoyu	Arane	Nori
Chinese Teas	Maple Syrup	Natural Spices	Dulse	Wasabi

Alkaline Nuts And Their Oils

Almonds	Hemp Hearts	Salba Seeds	Walnuts
Brazil	Hemp Seeds	Sesame Seeds, White	
Hazelnuts	Pumpkin Seeds	Sunflower Seeds	

Alkaline Forming Vegetables

Alfalfa	String	Red	Cucumber	Leeks	Sorrel
Almonds	Wax	White	Dandelion	Lettuce	Spinach
Artichokes	Beets	Green	Dill	Okra	Sprouts
Arugula	Bell Peppers	Carrots	Dock, Green	Olives	Squash
Asparagus	Orange	Celery	Eggplant	Onions	Sweet Potato
Avocados	Yellow	Cauliflower	Escarole	Parsley	Turnips
Bamboo	Red	Chard	Fennel	Peas	Watercress
Shoots	Broccoli	Chestnuts	Garlic	Pumpkin	White Potato
Beans	Brussels	Chicory	Kale	Radish	White Sweet
Green	Sprouts	Chives	Kohl Rabi	Rhubarb	Potato
Lima	Cabbage	Collards			Yams

The Road to Longevity
via a Healthy Mind, Body and Soul

People say to me, "how do you stay in such good shape…
I want to do whatever it is you're doing" That statement deserves
a multi-faceted response. I'll tell you what I do, then I'll make
some suggestions that I believe you can incorporate
into your own daily lives.

It is imperative that we stay active with the right exercise, eat healthy foods that work best within our bodies, keep our minds alert and our hearts in the right place. It is particularly urgent to be mindful of these things as we grow older in order to slow the aging process.

Of course, it is wonderful to have already built a strong healthy foundation that we can work to maintain. However, if we find that we have drifted away from these things over the years, it is still never too late to restart or begin a regimen of fitness, acuity of mind and proper eating habits. In other areas of the book I discuss diet more specifically, which is extremely important to how one looks and feels. In this section, however, I will focus on the powers of physical and mental exercise.

I often start my day by meditating for about half an hour. This practice eases me into the day ahead. Research has shown that meditation helps us relax and increases our capacity of concentration. Some neuroscientists have found that meditation shifts brain waves in the stress-receptive right lobe to the more serene-inclining left lobe. This shifting of the brain waves during meditation can enable a person raise their feelings of calmness.

My physical exercise program begins in the early morning with a 6 ½ mile run or, alternating daily, a 15 mile ride on my racing bike. Immediately after returning from the road, I jump into the pool and swim laps for a mile. I follow that with a peaceful, hour-long session of yoga that I do for the stretching exercise it provides me.

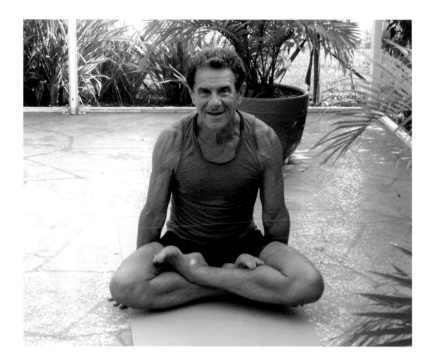

The exercise portion of my day ends in the late afternoon with a visit to the gym for weight training and strengthening for about an hour. I focus on various muscle groups, alternating them from day to day. Sometimes I work with a trainer; however, most of the time I work with the weight machines and free weights by myself.

This is the program that I adhere to five days a week. On weekends, I incorporate a number of these exercises, but I usually stagger them throughout the day. I also play an occasional game of tennis; not only is it fun, it provides a terrific aerobic workout. One other beneficial thing I take immense pleasure in is a long, leisurely walk on the beach to enjoy the splashing waves and ocean breezes, clear my head and count my blessings.

Let's not forget, one of the most important things you can do to rejuvenate your mind, body and soul is to get a good night's sleep. The general school of thought always was that everyone needed eight hours of sleep a night. Over the past number of years, however, a number of studies have shown that the hours of sleep need varies slightly from person to person. The one rule that I think we can all obey is to try to sleep for as many hours as it takes until your body feels like it has enough sleep. Our bodies do speak to us.

The discussion of a good night's sleep brings up the subject of a daytime mini sleep, commonly referred to as a "power nap". These naps are taken for a duration of not longer than twenty to thirty minutes. The short napping time allows you to feel refreshed without sleeping so long that you go into a normal sleep cycle without being able to complete it. If you do sleep too long, enter into a normal sleep cycle, then wake yourself, you can experience sleep inertia, in which you feel groggy, disoriented, and probably even sleepier than before beginning the nap.

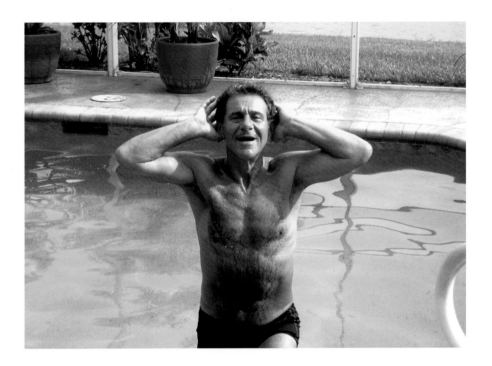

As yoga and meditation sometimes go hand in hand, I thought I would address both of those techniques for a moment. I mentioned earlier that I practice yoga for the stretching exercise it brings to my muscles. Yoga involves deliberate, structured breathing integrated with a series of postures. This technique produces a detoxifying effect on muscles and organs, resulting in a light yet strong body and improved circulation,

For years, I had one-on-one training sessions with professional yoga teachers and took group classes as well. During that time, I was able to learn, understand, and perfect the stances that felt good and worked for me. Now I enjoy my yoga sessions in the privacy of my own home. If you are not a practitioner of yoga, and you would like to try it, you can find tons of information and demonstrative help on the various disciplines through books, CDs, on-line websites, even on some cable TV channels. Keep yourself in check, and make sure that you are physically able to do these postures and stretches.

Meditation, like prayer, is something that can help center you if you open up to it. The physical act of meditation generally consists of simply sitting quietly, focusing on one's breathing or a word or phrase. As easy as that sounds, there are many people that just cannot get into a meditative state. My wife, for one, says that she cannot shut out her thoughts long enough to actually achieve that state. I have been practicing meditation for over 30 years, so I am able to enjoy its benefits. I say go for it; if it doesn't come along immediately, it's worth the practice. As with yoga, there are a multitude of places in which you can find information on meditating.

The best advice I can give anyone regarding physical activity is encompassed in one word: MOVE. Keeping active is beneficial to your entire body—muscle, bones, heart, lungs, and other organs—as well as to your mental and spiritual well-being.

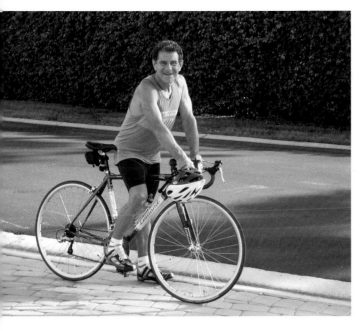

Walk. Simple as that; just walk. Take the dog for a walk. Take yourself around the block to start, then start expanding that block to two blocks, three, up to a mile, two miles, three, etc. If you have particularly inclement weather during parts of the year, go to a nearby mall and walk around it as many times as you like. Some malls even open their doors early for "mall walkers". Walk (or run) up and down the stairs.

Speed Walk or Run. Start slowly and build up; go at your own pace.

Dance. Around the house or out and about. In front of the mirror. Sing along; have fun with it.

Swim. Swimming is one of the best all-encompassing exercises you can do. It gives you a great aerobic workout and it moves all of your muscles, without putting undue compression on your joints and bones.

Bike. Whether you ride a regular bike or a speed bike, working your legs by pushing those pedals is a terrific way to strengthen your legs and back.

Pilates, stretching, yoga, calisthenics. All of these exercises are highly beneficial, each in their own way. Again, there are numerous places to find instructional information on these particular techniques.

Weight Training and Strengthening. Always start a weight training program under the supervision of a professional. While using weights can bring wonderful toning benefits, it is one of the modes of exercising that can hurt you if you are not careful or not completely aware of how you should be handling the equipment.

The Gym. Almost all of the exercise regimens outlined here can be done at home. If you do not have a pool, a Pilates ball, weights, etc., seek out your local gym. Not only can you find these things here, but you can also find professionals to help to learn and understand your personal exercise routine.

A final word on exercising. Make sure you are up to whatever it is you would like to do; if you've never done something before, do not jump into the middle of it. Start slowly, and with the OK from your health provider. Take guidance from your athletic professionals. They will help you set out a program that will be specific to your needs and goals.

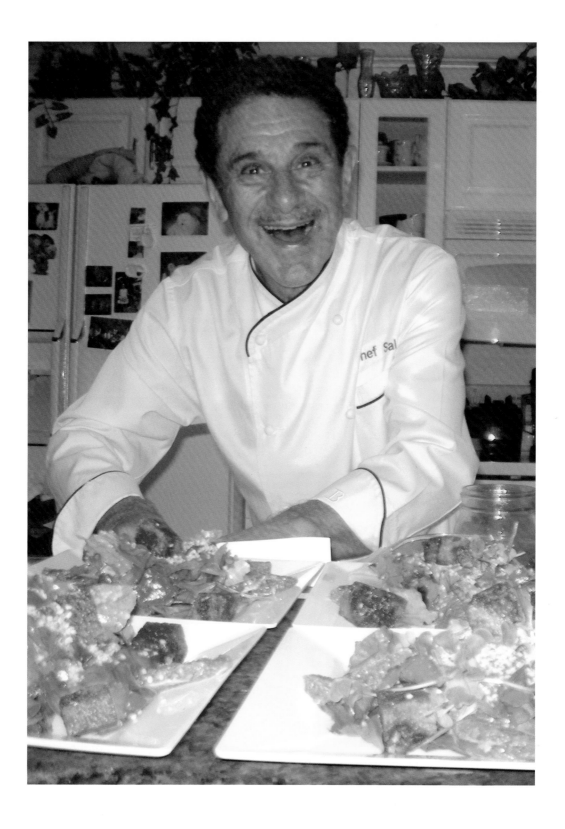

Around The Kitchen
Basic Information, Appliances and Tools

Raw cuisine preparation adapts many of the basics of cooked food, but does not use stoves, ovens, microwave ovens, toasters, grills, and the like. Raw cuisine is "cooked" at a very low temperature in multi-shelved dehydrators. Below is an overview of how a raw kitchen should be stocked and utilized.

SAFETY FIRST

Even with the proper tools in hand, it requires common sense to ensure that your kitchen is safe both for those who prepare it as well as for the diners who eat foods prepared in it. These rules are essential for a safe kitchen.

- Always wash your hands well with hot soapy water whenever moving to a new ingredient.

- Wash and sanitize your work station knives and cutting board whenever starting a project or moving to a new ingredient.

- Use a surface sanitizer or liquid germicide rather than using bleach for the same purpose. In high concentrations, bleach can be toxic.

- Whenever you do extensive cutting, place a wet flat cloth or non skid pad under your cutting board.

- Skilled knife work shows that the chef or cook takes pride in his or her work. The importance of the knives you use cannot be overemphasized. High quality, well made, and well maintained knives are fundamental. A list of knives I recommend that you have in your kitchen is found below. A sharp knife is a safe knife. Always keep a sharp edge on all of your knives. Never place knives in a sink filled with other items. If you reach into a sink filled with knives, forks, plates, etc., you will always find the knife first – whether you want to or not. If you knife is ever knocked out of your hand, or if you drop it, never try to catch it or keep it from falling. To do so is to invite injury.

You will add your own safety tips to this list, and I encourage you to do so. It is not meant to be comprehensive as much as it is intended to alert you to some of the things you need to think about as you prepare your meals.

APPLIANCES FOR USE IN RAW FOOD PREPARATION

There are four basic appliances that are mandatory for preparing raw food meals. There are quite a few brands on the market today for these appliances, all at varying price points. Although they all perform the same functions, some are better than others in speed, size, efficiency, etc. Do your homework; check out the brands that best fit your needs, and follow the manufacturers' guidelines. I'm noting the brands that I use in parentheses.

Dehydrator.

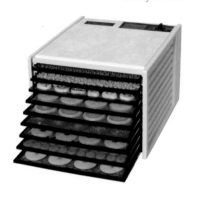

This is the appliance that "cooks" your food. Almost everything is dehydrated at 105°, occasionally up to 115°, to retain the integrity of the enzymes. Don't be shocked at the dehydrating times of some of these dishes. You may actually need to dehydrate some items for more than 30 hours. Dehydrators do not get hot, and can run for hours upon hours with little electricity expenditure. The dehydrator can also be used to warm up cold food items that just came out of the refrigerator. You have to closely monitor the warm up time, so that the product retains the consistency it had when it went in to be warmed. Nothing in it will burn, but foods could over-dehydrate to the point of becoming hard.

Food processor.

The food processor chops, slices, blends, grinds, etc. It comes with an assortment of blades that process foods in a variety of ways.

Juicer.

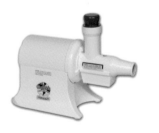

The juicer does exactly what its name implies. It allows you to put whole fruits or vegetables (after the obvious prep work, like removing pits) into the machine and coming away with fresh juice. The pulpy fiber is cast away from the juice and is stored for easy removal. The juice that you get from a juicer is quite different than putting a piece of fruit or vegetable into a blender or food processor. The latter two process the item, and a combination of fiber and juice remains as a thickened mixture.

Blender.

The blender does almost all of the things that a food processor does, except slicing and large dicing. However, it has the added ability to work with liquids in blending sauces, soups, beverages, etc. Often times the food processor and the blender are interchangeable in achieving a desired outcome.

BASIC UTENSILS

You most likely have some, most or all of the following utensils in your kitchen. Make sure that you do have these items at your disposal, because you will need all of them at one time or another.

- Sturdy cutting boards – both large and small. Wooden cutting boards are probably the safest to use in preparing fruits, vegetables, etc. If we were preparing any kind of meat or poultry, however, I would recommend against wood. You do not want to use plastic; glass is an option, but you run the risk of breakage. Just make sure that your wooden cutting boards are always kept clean.

- French knife, also known as a "chef's knife". The size of your chef's knife should be in proportion to the size of your hand. A six to eight inch blade is all you need if you have small hands. Those with larger hands may opt for a blade as long as ten inches.

- Paring knife. The familiar paring knife is indispensable for general use, as it is for small and delicate jobs.

- Mandoline. This is a terrific utensil that is used for thin slicing and cutting julienne strips. Mandolines often come with attachments for making other shapes, like a crinkle cut.

- Knife sharpener. Always keep a sharp edge on your knives.

- Vegetable peeler. Select a peeler that fits well in your hand and has a sharp precision blade.

- Strainers. Equip your kitchen with a large, sturdy strainer as well as a second, very fine strainer for straining sauces, purees and nut cheeses.

- Cheese cloth. Use alone or with strainers for an extremely fine-strained product.

- Hand grater. The best graters have several grating surfaces, allowing variations in how finely something is grated. Some graters also come with a sealed container into which the gratings are dropped, helping to keep your work station clean.

- Rubber spatulas. Choose spatulas that are both flexible and firm. Some less expensive rubber spatulas tend to be either too floppy or too rigid, avoid extremes.

- Stainless steel spatulas. These spatulas should be very thin; test the spatula in your hand. You will need a steel spatula to flip and turn food items, and you want them to feel easy to control.

- Squeezer for citrus fruits. Squeezers are different from juicers. There are both hand operated and electric squeezers. Their function is to ream a citrus fruit, one half at a time, to squeeze out all of the juice. There is no pulpy fiber left behind, just the rind of the fruit.

- Hand held mixer. A mixer is used in vessels where a blender or food processor cannot, allowing medium to high speed blending of foods contained in everything from a mixing bowl to a jar.

Working with and within the recipes in this book

The "Catch-All" Drawer

"Ahhh, this porridge is just right."
~ Goldilocks

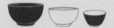

There are 126 recipes in this book. I have developed, prepared, tested, tasted, shared and served all of them. My goal was to assemble a set of recipes that would be easy to understand, simple to prepare, filled with quality nutritional alkaline food products, and finally to duplicate that happy, contented Goldilocks taste experience.

Found in kitchens everywhere is the infamous "junk" drawer, or the more palatable "catch-all" drawer. You know what I'm talking about. This chapter, metaphorically speaking, is the catch-all drawer of this book.

It contains information to help you prepare the recipes found here. For instance, there are a number of ingredients that I use throughout the book that may be interchanged to create a taste that you prefer. Although I developed these recipes to achieve the flavor impact I envisioned, there is enough wiggle room for adaptation.

The recipes in this book can be doubled, halved, tripled, etc. The chapter of "appetizers and entrees" is filled with recipes that can be used to make small portions (appetizers) or larger portions (entrées) of the same dish. That also applies for salads; they can be made as a side dish salad or an entrée salad. It's just a matter of portion size.

I have included some basic helpful hints that I use in my kitchen, ranging from storage containers to explaining the difference between a large dice and a brunoise cut. So, if you're looking for something in other areas of this book, and can't find it, plow through this chapter.

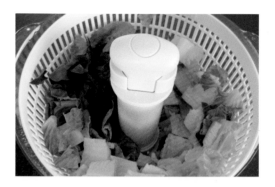
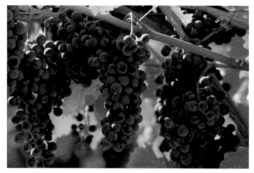
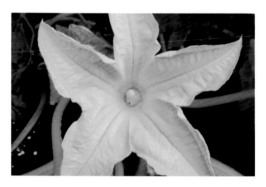
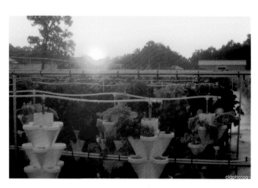

- FOOD CLEANLINESS. Properly wash all of your food. I thoroughly wash (including soaking) all my fruits and vegetables in a solution of water mixed with a few drops of food-grade peroxide. Rinse everything and dry. A salad spinner is perfect for getting rid of the excess solution.

- SALT. Unless otherwise specified, I use the pink Himalayan sea salt in my recipes that call for salt. Some of the recipes simply indicate "sea salt", or even just "salt"; either of those terms indicate Himalayan sea salt, however. There are a few other salts you might like to try. Herbamare is an herb flavored salt that is ground into something more like a powder. Himalayan black crystal salt, otherwise known as "kala namak" comes in a variety of grinds, from course to fine powder. It has an almost sweet taste and is great for use in garnishing soups and salads. It does have a tendency to dissolve when it touches moisture, so it should be used just prior to serving if used as a garnish. If used within the recipe, it will darken the food product slightly. Smoked apple Himalayan sea salt has a very interesting flavor. The key word here is "smoked"; you could add a touch of this salt into meat substitute recipes like kebobs or burgers to achieve a grilled flavor. But be ultra careful with it – it is very salty and has an extremely strong smoky flavor. I would recommend tasting just the smallest pinch of this salt to gauge how much you'd like to use.

- STORAGE. Store all of your soups, sauces, leftovers, nuts – everything – in glass containers. Plastic has the ability to leach out into your foods.

- ROASTING. Roasting vegetables is extremely easy. There are a few variables to consider, however. Are the vegetables fresh or frozen? What is the desired outcome of the roasted flavor? Start with the vegetable itself. If fresh, prepare in the manner in which you choose to serve it—peel, core, seed, slice, chop, etc. If frozen, allow to thaw at room temperature or thaw in a shallow bowl of water placed in the bottom of the dehydrator. When vegetables are prepared to your liking, coat lightly with grape seed oil and flavor with garlic powder, onion powder and sea salt. If you wish to go beyond the simple seasonings, you can add in any number of minced herbs, pepper and/or substitute plain sea salt with a flavored salt. Place on Teflex sheets and dehydrate for about 3 ½ hours until roasted but still aldente, or to your liking. Certain vegetables may require a longer dehydrating time than others. If you plan to mix a variety of vegetables, cook each to your desired liking, then mix together to serve. See ABCs of Roasting Vegetables in the Appetizer/Entrée Recipe section of this book.

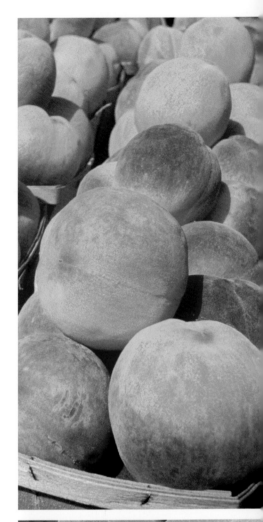

- SWEETENERS. Agave is my prime sweetener, with an occasional use of maple syrup. There are a number of sweetening products on the market, including coconut palm sugar, that are quite nutritious. Test them out; they come with their own flavor and texture profiles.

- OILS. Speaking of oils, my oil of choice is grape seed oil; recipes that indicate only "oil" should incorporate grape seed. I prefer this type of oil for its ability to add viscosity to a recipe without adding flavor. There are recipes here in which I indicate extra virgin olive oil or others. You can always substitute oils for flavor enhancements. In the chapter regarding alkaline foods, there is a list of oils from which you may choose to use. Some of the other oils that I have specified are red palm oil, Salba oil, avocado oil, sesame oil, etc.

- FRUITS AND VEGETABLES. They are meant to be eaten ripe; unripe foods do not carry their total capacity of enzymes, and it is difficult to digest. If you buy items that are not ripe (mostly fruits), ripen them in one of two ways. For larger items like pineapple and papaya, let them sit out in the sun if it is warm; if it is cold outside, place them in a win-

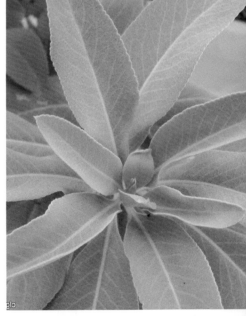

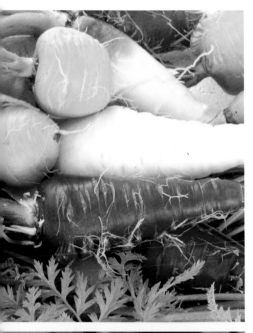

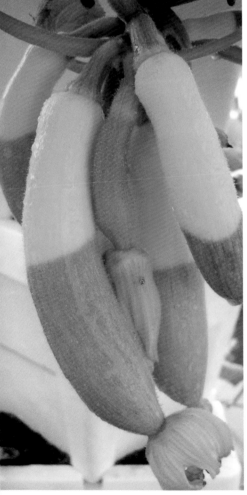

dow in order that they receive the sun's rays through the glass. For smaller items like pears, nectarines, avocadoes, etc., place them into a brown paper bag for a day or two. The bag acts like an incubator in a way; the food items release a natural hormone gas called ethylene. That ethylene, trapped inside the bag, will ripen the food.

- FRESH HERBS. One of the nicest things that you can do for yourself and your kitchen is to grown herbs in pots near a window. You will always have fresh herbs on hand, and your kitchen will smell great.

- SNACKS. Make batches of snacks found in the chapters on "bites" and "beverages; store in glass containers in your refrigerator, and use whenever you just feel like noshing. The nuts and crackers have a relatively long shelf line; however the beverages should be consumed within a day or so.

- HEATING. Raw soups can be warmed by the heat generated by the blender during preparation, by pouring the soup in a bowl and placing it onto the bottom of the dehydrator or by warming the bowl alone in the dehydrator. A short time in the dehydrator can also warm anything that comes right out of the refrigerator to take off the chill. You have to be vigilant in your timing; too long in the dehydrator could alter the consistency of a solid food item. Usually 15 minutes or less at 105° will do the trick.

- CLEAN-PREP CHESTNUTS. Chestnuts have a bitter, dark skin. To use, wash the nut well; remove any dark skin.

- JAPANESE VEGETABLES. Although these vegetables are listed on the alkaline foods list, it is important to know that these tasty products are filled with enzymes, minerals and vitamins. A partial list includes dulse, arame, edamame, nori, wakeme, etc.

- ICE CREAM. You may enjoy any of the ice creams found in this book directly from a bowl, rolled into balls and coated with shredded coconut or minced nuts and refrozen, like a bon-bon, or put into a popsicle mold to create a frosty treat on a stick.

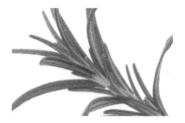  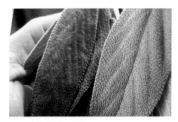

- KNIFE SKILLS. Proper paring and dicing. The proper way to hold a knife while preparing food is to grasp the blade firmly between the pad of your hand, your thumb, and the knuckle of your index finger just in front of the bolster, curling your remaining fingers around the bottom of the handle. Some of the various cuts referred to in the recipes are:

- LARGE DICE. Cut into squares ¾ x ¾ x ¾ inches.

- MEDIUM DICE. Cut into squares ½ x ½ x ½ inches.

- SMALL DICE. Cut into squares ¼ x ¼ x ¼ inches.

- RONDELLE. A coin shaped cut, achieved by slicing carrots, parsnips, etc. across the body of the fruit or vegetable.

- JULIENNE. Cut into long thin strips, ⅛ x ⅛ x 2½ inches.

- MINCED. Chopped into very tiny pieces, or squeezed through a garlic press.

- BRUNOISE. This cut is a shorter, squarer version of a Julienne; it is ⅛ x ⅛ x ⅛ inches; the same thickness and width of the julienne, but only ⅛ inch long.

- SHREDDED OR GRATED. As the word implies, these food products are run over a shredder or a grater to achieve very thin, and/or very small pieces.

- ZEST. The smallest shreds and pieces are achieved by running the food item (only the rind) over the smallest grating utensil.

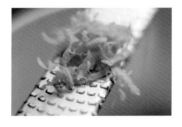 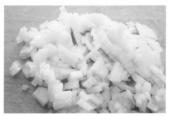 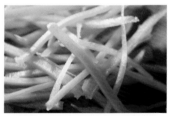

"We are indeed much more than what we eat, but what we eat can nevertheless help us to be much more than what we are."

– Adelle Davis (1904-1974)
American author and pioneer in the fledgling field of nutrition during the mid-20th century.

- **BELL'S SEASONING.** Bell's has been the go-to seasoning for poultry in homes across the United States, and most people associate it with the turkey flavoring for Thanksgiving dinner. However, this distinctly American seasoning comes from herbs grown around the world.. Spain, Portugal, Greece, Mexico, Yugoslavia, Albania, Nigeria, France, Peru and India. It is free of salt, sugar preservatives, artificial coloring and additives. Bell's Seasoning is a natural product; you may choose to use it or make your own with fresh organics. Below is a compilation of the amount of the herbs (and pepper) that replicates Bell's Seasoning extremely well. Mince or grate and combine all of the ingredients and store in a jar in the refrigerator.

1 tbsp rosemary	1 tsp thyme
1 ½ tsp oregano	½ tsp marjoram
1 ½ tsp sage	¼ tsp pepper
1 ½ tsp ginger	

- **GARAM MASALA.** Garam masala is a Hindi description, meaning "hot mixture". It is a basic blend of ground spices common in Indian and other South Asian cuisines. It is used alone or with other seasonings. Garam masala is pungent, but not "hot" in the same way as is a chili pepper. You can find organic garam masala in stores, but if you wish to make your own, follow the list of ingredients, and their amounts. Mix them all together; place in a glass container and store in a cool, dry place.

1 tbsp ground cumin	1 tsp ground cinnamon
1 ½ tsp ground coriander	½ tsp ground cloves
1 ½ tsp ground cardamom	½ tsp ground nutmeg
1 ½ tsp ground pepper	

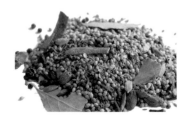
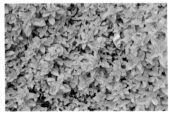
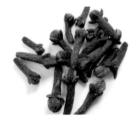

Odd Duck Ingredients

What They Are...

What's Good About Them...

Where to Buy Them...

What the heck is this?

I've never heard of it!

There are a number of ingredients in this book that you may never have run across before. Some of them were new to me as well when I began my journey into raw alkaline cuisine. I will do my best to convey the information I have on these items. You will probably be able to find them all at your local organic health food store, but in case your store does not carry any particular item, I have included web sites from which you may purchase them.

Flax

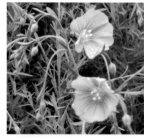

A slender, annual plant with beautiful blue flowers, flax produces a small and shiny brown seed that is slightly larger than a sesame seed. Flax has been known and utilized since the Stone Ages, originating in Mesopotamia. Although initially cultivated for its fiber (which was woven into threads and fabrics and famously used by the Egyptians), the first records of flax's culinary use stems from ancient Greece, where its health benefits were widely praised. Flaxseed continues to be enjoyed and easily incorporated into foods in the modern world, and is most nutritiously assimilated when ground.

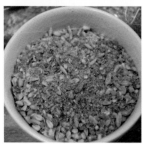

Flaxseeds are best known for their healthy essential fatty acid profile, and boast the highest source of omega 3's of any plant-based food. These "EFAs" are known to have a number of advantages, including promoting a healthy cardiovascular and immune system. Additionally, flaxseed is rich in lignans, which are known to balance hormone levels, and the seeds also serve as a fantastic source of soluble fiber. Just by sprinkling it into various foods, flax power is an easy way to fortify any recipe with its naturally occurring nutrients and mild nutty flavor. May be obtained on line through www.navitasnaturals.com.

Goji Berries

Goji berries have been appreciated in Asian herbal medicine for several millenniums, but only recently have western cultures "discovered" the power of this remarkable food. A small red berry, gojis are indigenous to the Himalayan mountain range.

The goji berry has long been regarded as one of the most nutrient-rich superfoods on the planet, with ancient Chinese monks crediting this berry to greater health, vitality, longevity, energy, and stamina. Western science agrees that indeed this special berry has a remarkable nutritional profile, and it is now among the most highly sought-after superfoods around.

Arguably among the most potent superfoods known, the goji berry offers an exceptional balance of daily macronutrients: containing carbohydrates, high-quality protein, healthy fat, and soluble fiber. The goji's solid plant-based protein is packed with 18 amino acids – including all 8 essential amino acids – which is 10% of the fruits composition. Also full of free-radical-devouring antioxidants, goji berries have been historically used to support the immune system and longevity. Rich in vitamin A and a good source of vitamin C, these berries additionally possess over 20 trace minerals and vitamins including zinc, iron, phosphorus, riboflavin (B2), vitamin E, and carotenoids which include beta-carotene. And to put things in perspective on just how powerful the little goji berry is, ounce per ounce it contains more vitamin C than oranges, more beta carotene than carrots, and more iron than spinach.

With a chewy texture and a pleasant taste somewhere in between a dried cherry and a cranberry, goji berries make a nutritious replacement for raisins or dried fruit. May be obtained on line through www.navitasnaturals.com.

Hemp

The hemp plant is native to Asia but cultivated in many parts of the world. It is the source of a nutritious, edible seed (hemp seed). Hemp is one of the earliest known plants to be cultivated by humans, with a recorded history of over 12,000 years, and has since been grown all around the world for food. An immensely sustainable crop, hemp's nutritional benefits are highly renowned, and the hemp seed legacy continues as an ideal source of fuel for human health and energy. The heart of the seed is the most potent of the plant.

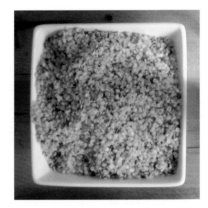

Though it may be just a small seed, hemp offers a huge nutritional content. Hemp seeds are naturally a fantastic protein source: they contain all of the essential amino acids, are highly digestible, and are one of the highest sources of complete protein of all plant-based foods. Hemp also has a very well-balanced ratio of essential fatty acids (EFAs) – Omega 3, 6, and 9 – which are excellent for cardiovascular health and promote a strong immune system (among many other benefits). A great source of dietary fiber, magnesium, iron, zinc, and potassium, hemp is a true super seed.

A soft nut, the shelled hemp tastes reminiscent of a sunflower seed, with a distinctive richness. Enjoy hemp seeds by themselves, or try them sprinkled on just about anything, including nut cheeses, salads, soups, dips, or baked into recipes. Hemp protein has a mild taste, which becomes a background flavor when combined with other ingredients. Just a spoonful or two of it is the perfect protein boost when added to a dish. May be obtained on line through www.navitasnaturals.com.

Lucuma Powder

Lucuma is considered a healthy alternative sweetener as it lends a sweet taste to recipes, but is very low in sugars. With naturally occurring beta-carotene, niacin, and iron, lucuma powder is a welcome antidote to notorious "empty calorie" sweeteners.

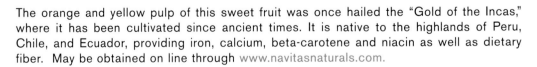

Lucuma powder has a distinctively sweet fragrance and full-bodied, maple-like taste. A deliciously versatile dessert ingredient, lucuma blends well to make alluring smoothies, puddings, and ice creams.

The orange and yellow pulp of this sweet fruit was once hailed the "Gold of the Incas," where it has been cultivated since ancient times. It is native to the highlands of Peru, Chile, and Ecuador, providing iron, calcium, beta-carotene and niacin as well as dietary fiber. May be obtained on line through www.navitasnaturals.com.

Maca

The root of the maca plant has been used in Andean cultures as a source of nourishment and healing for many millenniums. A radish-like root, maca is indigenous to the Peruvian highlands. The harvested root of the maca plant was traditionally used by Incan warriors in preparation for difficult expositions and battles, and was consumed to increase stamina and energy. Maca is considered to be one of the most appreciated superfoods on the market.

Maca has long been used to increase stamina and combat fatigue; the root is a superb adaptogen, as it enables the body to more easily adapt to and regulate stress factors imposed upon it. Studies have also identified four alkaloids present in maca, which are known to nourish the endocrine system (the system in the body which is responsible for the production and maintenance of hormones). Maca root is a highly nutrient-dense whole food, as it is packed with vitamins, plant sterols, many essential minerals, amino acids and healthy fats. This is a particularly powerful and balanced food for athletes and those who are looking to combat stress or increase stamina.

Maca has an earthy taste that is mildly nutty with a hint of butterscotch; it is easily blended into superfood smoothies, various plant-based milks, chocolate or other dessert recipes. May be obtained on line through www.navitasnaturals.com.

Mesquite

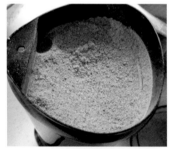

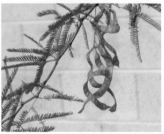

Mesquite is a traditional staple food of indigenous cultures from the arid regions of the Americas. Native to South America, the mesquite tree produces large seed-filled pods, which are collected, ground into flour, and used in recipes. Desert dwellers often relied upon the sweet pods as a staple food, and would even use them as a bartering tool with neighboring tribes. Today, mesquite's distinct flavor and wonderful smell continue to be enjoyed in many culinary applications, with its health benefits widely respected.

Mesquite is of particularly great value to those looking to balance blood sugar levels. Mesquite flour offers a naturally sweet flavor to recipes, but its sugars are derived from fructose (which does not require insulin to digest and is readily metabolized). Additionally, the flour is an excellent form of fiber – meeting almost a quarter of daily needs in just two tablespoons – which not only improves digestion but further benefits sugar metabolism. Mesquite also contains lysine (an amino acid), as well as notable quantities of digestible protein, calcium, magnesium, potassium, iron and zinc.

Mesquite powder has a sweet, smoky flavor that is similar to carob, with caramel undertones. Its rich taste and aroma pairs well with both vanilla and chocolate. Mesquite blends beautifully with coconut or almond milk, is an excellent addition to smoothies, and is fantastic dishes. when sprinkled into ice cream. Mesquite is low glycemic and is low in fat and carbs. May be obtained on line through www.navitasnaturals.com.

Arame (Arami)

The most mild tasting of all Japanese sea vegetables, it is hand harvested in the wild, shredded and naturally air dried. It is versatile and easy to prepare. Arame is rich in dietary fiber, low calorie, low sodium, and a good source of vitamin A, calcium, and magnesium. It is great in salads and soups.

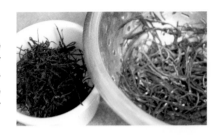

Daikon (Radish)

The daikon radish is a long cylindrical white root, shaped much like a carrot. Raw daikon is used to aid in digestion. Laboratory analysis has shown that the juice of raw daikon is abundant in digestive enzymes similar to those found in the human digestive tract. These enzymes help transform complex carbohydrates, fats, and proteins into their matching components. Traditional Japanese diets use daikon to help digest oils, and help digest the protein. Grated daikon is a wonderful aid to people with a weak digestive system.

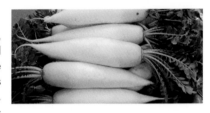

At Tokyo's College of Pharmacy, researchers have discovered that daikon juice actually inhibits the formation of dangerous chemicals in the body. Nitrosamines, a type of carcinogen, can form in the stomach from chemicals present in both natural and processed foods. Daikon juice contains substances identified as "phenolic compounds" that can block this potentially dangerous reaction. Thus, a diet including raw daikon may help to reduce the risk of cancer.

Daikon has also been shown to be effective as a diuretic and decongestant. As a diuretic, raw daikon promotes the discharge of excess water by the kidneys. The result is increased urination and gradual reduction of the swelling condition known as edema. As a decongestant, the enzymes in daikon juice seem to help dissolve mucus and phlegm in the respiratory system and facilitate their discharge from the body. It is a powerful cleanser with high water content and special enzymes that fortify the liver and aid in detoxifying the digestive tract.

Hiziki (Hijiki)

Hiziki is a wild Japanese sea vegetable hand harvested from waters off eastern Japan, then naturally sun dried. It is one of the most mineral rich sea vegetables. Hiziki is full of delicious, bold, sweet, concentrated nourishment. It is low calorie, fat free, rich in dietary fiber, and a good source of vitamin B2, calcium and magnesium.

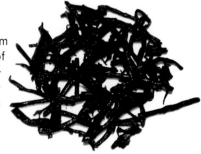

Nori

Nori is a seaweed with a mildly sweet, salty taste that is usually dried, and originating in Japanese cuisine. Nori is the Japanese name for a delectable red seaweed that grows in the country's surrounding waters. With celebrated culinary use reported back to the 8th century, Nori has never wavered in its reign as Japan's most popular sea vegetable — best known for its role as a wrapper around sushi. Once harvested, raw fronds are pressed into thin sheets, a process originating from the ancient art of Japanese papermaking. The resulting delicacy is ready to be enjoyed in all kinds of savory cuisine.

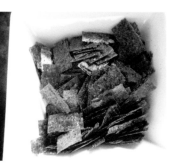

Nori is a low calorie superfood overflowing with bioavailable nutrients. Grown in the Sea of Japan, nori contains almost 50% protein — the highest of any seaweed. Saturated with minerals (including ten times more calcium and iron than dairy products, ounce per ounce), and hosting a wide spectrum of bioavailable vitamins, antioxidants, and lignans, nori serves as a nutrient-dense ingredient.

Wakame

Wakame is a brownish-green seaweed, having large fronds which grow in clusters. and traditionally dried for use in soups, salads, and side dishes. It is one of the most hearty vegetables of the sea, used in Japanese, Chinese, and Korean cuisine as an important health food It has also been a key component of Eastern medicine for centuries.

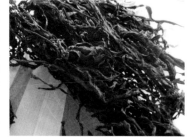

Wakame's salty taste is not simply "salt"; it is a balanced combination of essential organic minerals including iron, calcium, and magnesium, alongside valuable trace minerals. Additionally, wakame is well known for its detoxifying antioxidants, Omega 3 fatty acids and body-building vegetable proteins. Wakame also provides many vitamins like vitamin C and much of the B spectrum, and serves as an excellent source of both soluble and insoluble fiber.

Dried wakame makes a highly nutritious and flavorful cooking ingredient, imparting a satisfying sea-salty flavor to savory recipes. The seaweed is easily rehydrated with water, expanding slightly and becoming tender after soaking. Wakame is most widely known for its role as a featured ingredient in health-promoting miso soup. However, wakame may also be used in a variety of other soups, blended into sauces and nutritious salads.

Wasabi

One Japanese food that has some surprising health benefits is wasabi. Wasabi is a root vegetable often ground into a paste and served as a sauce in sushi restaurants. What are the health benefits of wasabi?

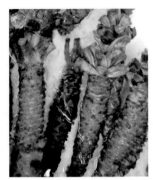

Wasabi is a rich source of chemicals known as isothiocyanates. These are the same anti-cancer chemicals found in broccoli and cabbage. These isothiocyanates appear to activate enzymes in the liver which detoxify cancer causing substances before they can do damage to the body. They also appear to interfere with other steps in the formation and metastasis of cancer cells. More importantly, they exert their anti-cancer effects without damaging normal cells.

The same isothiocyanates that give wasabi its cancer fighting capabilities also help to reduce inflammation by preventing platelet application. Researchers hope that wasabi may be used in the future to fight inflammation associated with such diseases as arthritis, asthma, and allergic reactions. More research is needed in this area. Because wasabi inhibits platelet aggregation, it's thought that it may reduce the risk of heart attack and stroke by preventing abnormal clot formation.

Not only does wasabi appear to prevent inflammation, growth of tumors, and abnormal platelet clumping, it also has anti-bacterial properties. One study demonstrated its ability to stop the growth of certain strains of bacteria that cause food poisoning. So convincing is the evidence that companies have already started making wasabi based antibacterial hand washes. It's also thought that wasabi can kill the bacteria that cause dental problems. To get the health benefits of wasabi, be sure you're buying the real thing.

If any of the above Japanese vegetables are not available at your local organic health food store or Asian market, they may all (with the possible exception of raw Daikon) be obtained on line through www.edenfoods.com or www.asianfoodgrocer.com.

Irish Moss

Among the many foods that are considered to be super foods, Irish Moss is a lesser known item. Irish moss is a species of seaweed, that grows in massive amounts in the rocky parts of the Atlantic coasts of America and Europe. It also is found in parts of the Pacific. It gets its name because it's most abundant near Ireland. When it's fresh, Irish moss is soft and varies in color. This seaweed is used in foods such as jellies and gelatin. The gelatin can go into ice creams, drinks, and other deserts. There are many health benefits of Irish moss.

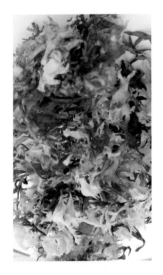

The seaweed can help protect against arteriosclerosis, hyper tension, and fat buildup. It can also help prevent the buildup of cholesterol, and protect against obesity. It helps to increase metabolism which can lead to the ability to burn off fat quicker.

Irish Moss continued on next page

By helping to prevent these problems, Irish moss can help lower your risk of heart attack and stroke.

Irish moss is an expectorant, meaning it can break up mucus and help clear out the lungs of any phlegm that builds up with a common cold. Because of the expectorant qualities, Irish moss helps to prevent a common cold from turning into pneumonia. Irish moss can treat other respiratory problems such as bronchitis.

Irish moss has been found to be very helpful with the recovery of radiation poisoning and cancer. This is due to the plant's high iodine content. Iodine is difficult to come by, and is found mainly in table salt. People don't get as much iodine in their diets as they should, so Irish moss is beneficial for that purpose alone. Along with iodine, Irish moss also contains calcium, sulfur, potassium, and vitamin E.   You can purchase Irish Moss at www.livingtreecommunity.com.

Longanberries

Longanberries are not to be confused with Loganberries; they have a taste very similar to the lychee. The Longanberry has a nickname, Dragon Eye, because when you open up the shell of a longanberry, you'll see a filmy and liquidy jelly, and inside of that round jelly you'll be able to see a black seed that is similar to a pupil of an eye. The longanberry itself is round and about one inch in diameter. They grow on trees that are usually found around Southeast Asia, but a number of farms in North America are now growing the trees and harvesting the fruit. The berries can be used in soups, desserts or snacks. Longanberries have been used through many years as an herbal medicine. They are rich in Vitamins A and C and contain the B vitamins, iron, magnesium, potassium, and a host of other minerals. Loganberries are a seasonal fruit; if your organic health food store does not carry them, try local farms or–if needed–substitute lychee.

Nama Shoyu

No other soy sauce in America comes close to this 100% organic, non-GMO Nama Shoyu in flavor or quality. It's the only soy sauce that's aged for four years in cedar kegs by a unique double-brew process, so it can be made with less salt naturally, while still retaining its full-bodied flavor and delicate bouquet. Nama Shoyu is also unpasteurized (the only raw soy sauce available in North America); it's full of health-giving live enzymes and beneficial organisms like lactobacillus.

Although I try to use raw, organic Nama Shoyu sparingly, I recognize that it is an essential ingredient for a lot of savory (and even some sweet) raw organic dishes–it gives them that extra taste that nothing else can deliver. Nama Shoyu is manufactured by Ohsawa, a macrobiotics-producing company; it is available just about everywhere. You can also order it on line at www.mothernature.com if you cannot find it in your store.

Appetizers and Entrées

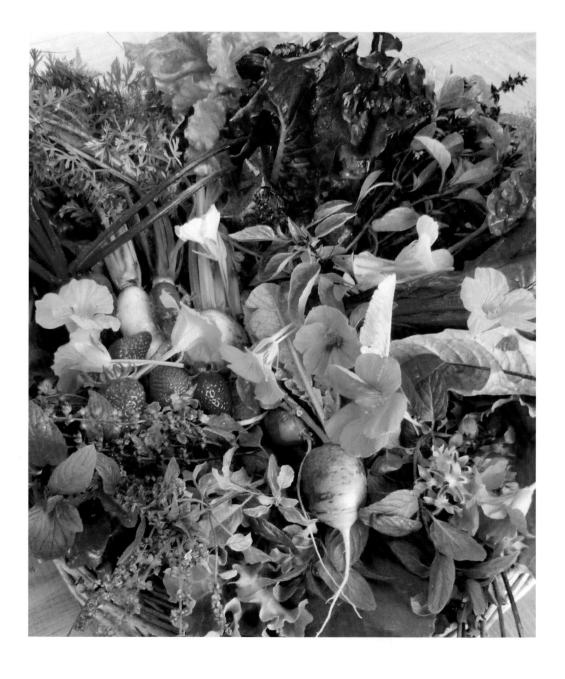

ABCs of Roasting Vegetables

INGREDIENTS

simple seasoning

grape seed oil

garlic powder

onion powder

Himalayan sea salt

FLAVOR-SPECIFIC SEASONING

variety of fresh herbs, fine chopped

ground black pepper

Herbamare salt, or other flavored salt, as substitute for plain sea salt

PREPARATION INSTRUCTIONS

Roasting vegetables is extremely easy. There are a few variables to consider, however. Are the vegetables fresh or frozen? What is the desired outcome of the roasted flavor?

Start with the vegetable itself. If fresh, prepare in the manner in which you choose to serve it – peel, core, seed, slice, chop, etc. If frozen, allow to thaw at room temperature or thaw in a shallow bowl of water placed in the bottom of the dehydrator.

When vegetables are prepared to your liking, coat lightly with grape seed oil and flavor with garlic powder, onion powder and sea salt. If you wish to go beyond the simple seasonings, you can add in any number of minced herbs, pepper and/or substitute plain sea salt with a flavored salt.

Place on Teflex sheets and dehydrate for about 3½ hours until roasted but still al dente, or to your liking. Certain vegetables may require a longer dehydrating time than others.

If you plan to mix a variety of vegetables, cook each to your desired liking, then mix together to serve.

Amazing Veggie Burger

INGREDIENTS

8 ounces walnuts, washed well, dried

8 ounces carrots, peeled, large diced

½ bunch fresh parsley, washed well, without stems

½ cup sweet potato, peeled and diced

1 stalk celery, diced

2 garlic cloves

assorted fresh herbs

touch cayenne powder

1 tbsp nutritional yeast

⅓ cup olive oil

1½ tsp onion powder

1½ tsp cumin powder

juice of 1 lemon

*1 tbsp nama shoyu

salt and black pepper to taste

*For less sodium, use raw coconut aminos

PREPARATION INSTRUCTIONS

1) Crush walnuts in food processor; set aside in large bowl.

2) Crush carrots in food processor; add to bowl with walnuts

3) Add sweet potato, parsley, celery, and garlic to food processor; chop until very coarse.

4) Place mixture in same bowl as walnuts and carrots. Blend everything together well.

5) Add lemon juice, olive oil, nutritional yeast, cumin powder, cayenne, onion powder and nama shoyu. Salt and pepper to taste.

6) Make patties and put on Teflon sheets or plastic wrap and dehydrate for 4 hours at 105°.

7) Turn patties over; dehydrate for 7 more hours.

8) Drizzle burgers with Avocado Dressing (see recipe page ?).

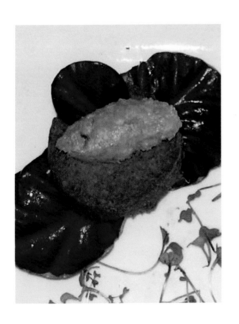

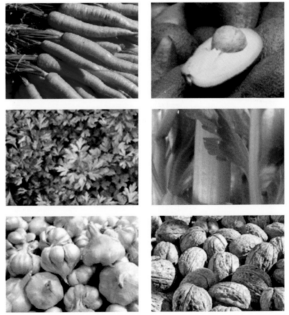

Dinner Loaf with Basil Pesto

INGREDIENTS

¾ cup sunflower seeds soaked 3 hours, drain and dry

¾ cup flaxseed, soak 3 hours, drain and dry

¾ cup raw almonds, soak 6 hours, drain and dry

½ cup celery juice

½ cup carrots, finely grated

1 tbsp cumin powder

½ cup nama shoyu

¼ tsp cayenne powder

5 cloves minced garlic

½ cup grape seed oil

½ yellow onion, diced

1 cup diced celery

PREPARATION INSTRUCTIONS

1) Process nuts and seeds in blender, until meal consistency is achieved. Mince onion, garlic and celery and finely shred carrots.

2) Add all ingredients in a bowl and mix thoroughly. Add the seed/nut mixture and all other ingredients (except the celery juice and grape seed oil) together in the blender. (The nuts won't blend well without liquid.) Make sure to break apart any lumps.

3) Spread the mixture evenly on Teflex sheet to thickness of about 1 inch. Dehydrate at 105° for about 10 hours. Flip the tray over onto an empty tray, and gently peel the Teflex sheet off the loaf. Return to the dehydrator for another 20 hours.

4) Serve with basil walnut pesto.

Italian Drops "Meatballs"

INGREDIENTS

½ cup walnuts, soaked for 1 hour, well washed and dried

2 ounces raisins, soaked for 20 minutes and dried

2 tsp fresh garlic, peeled, diced

2 ounces carrots, peeled, large diced

½ tsp nama shoyu

1 tbsp red palm oil

1 tsp dried basil

1½ tsp dried Italian herbs

⅛ tsp dried red pepper flakes

1 tbsp ground Salba seeds

1 tsp onion powder

1 tsp Himalayan sea salt

PREPARATION INSTRUCTIONS

1) Put all ingredients in food processor (except Salba seeds and oils); chop till well mixed.

2) Slowly blend in oils; add Salba seeds and blend all together well.

3) Roll into small balls and place on Teflex sheet. Dehydrate at 110° for 13 hours, turning after 6 hours.

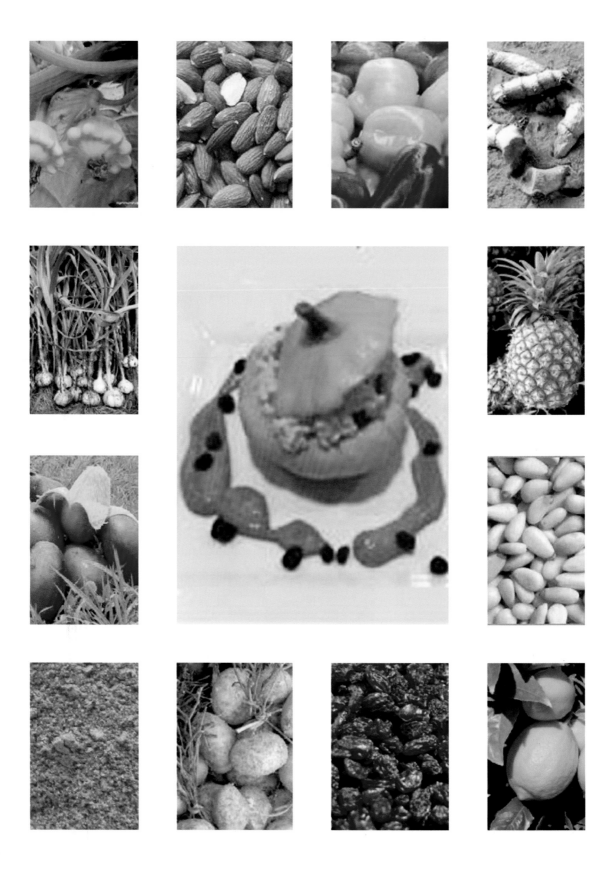

Jicama Couscous Filled Patty Pan Squash with Essence of Mango and Bell Pepper

INGREDIENTS

6 to 8 patty pan squash

3 cups jicama

1 cup pine nuts

2 tbsp Salba oil

2 tbsp nutritional yeast

1 tsp garlic powder

¼ tsp turmeric

~~ cayenne to taste

~~ sea salt to taste

PREPARATION INSTRUCTIONS

1) Cut and remove tops from patty pan squash. Scrape out insides, being careful not to puncture a hole in the squash.

2) Pour a small amount of sea salt-infused water into squash "bowl"; place on Teflex sheet and dehydrate for about 8 hours or until al dente.

3) Peel and dice jicama.

4) Place jicama and pine nuts into food processor and process until very fine.

5) Add remaining ingredients into processor and blend well.

6) Put mixture into strainer and remove as much liquid as possible.

7) Fill each patty pan squash with couscous mixture.

8) Ladle mango and bell pepper essence around squash "bowls".

9) Garnish with plumped raisins.

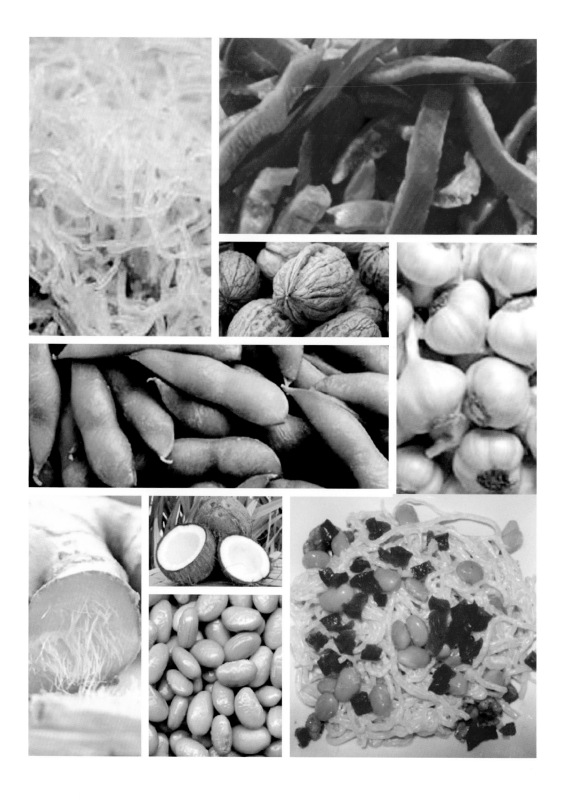

Kelp Noodle Swirl of Edamame, Brunoise of Red Pepper, Asian Ginger Emulsion, Garnished with Crunchy Cinnamon Walnuts

INGREDIENTS

MAIN DISH

4 ounces kelp noodles per person, thoroughly rinsed, dried and cut into desired lengths

~ shelled edamame beans

~ brunoise cut red pepper, dehydrated on Teflex sheet for 30 minutes

ASIAN GINGER EMULSION

1 tbs white miso

2 cloves peeled garlic

1 tsp rice wine vinegar

2 tbs apple cider vinegar

1 tbs fresh ginger, peeled and diced

1 tbs maple syrup

1 tsp Himalayan sea salt

1/3 cup grape seed oil

1 tbs sesame oil

1 tbs sesame tahini

1 tsp raw coconut aminos

1 tbs cold water

~ cayenne to taste

PREPARATION INSTRUCTIONS

1) In a large bowl, toss together the kelp noodles, shelled edamame beans and brunoise-cut red pepper. Set aside.

2) Put all emulsion ingredients in blender, except sesame oil, grape seed oil, and water.

3) Blend on high speed; when all ingredients are well blended, finish by adding all oils, and dilute with cold water.

4) Pour emulsion over the kelp noodle/ edamame/red pepper mixture and toss until everything is coated with the emulsion.

5) Portion out the mixture onto individual plates; decorate with crunchy cinnamon walnuts and some fresh black pepper to taste.

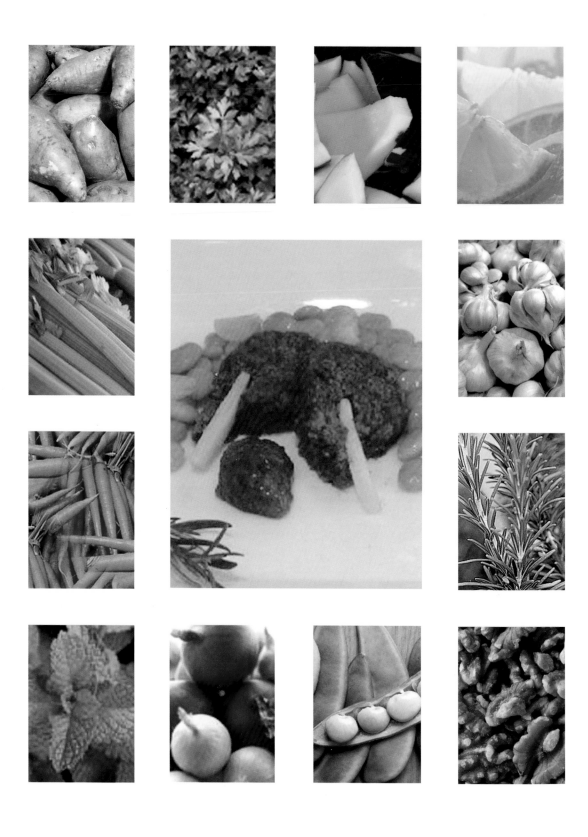

Lamb Chop Served with Spicy Mint Jelly Sauce

INGREDIENTS

¼ cup sweet potato, peeled, diced

1 cup celery stalk, diced

½ cup carrots, peeled, large diced

½ cup walnuts, washed well, dried

1 garlic clove

1 tsp onion powder

¼ bunch fresh parsley, washed well, dried

½ cup grape seed oil

½ lemon, juiced

1 tbsp nama shoyu

1 tbsp adobo seasoning

1 tbsp fresh rosemary, small diced

~~ cayenne and sea salt to taste

1 Asian pear cut into thick julienne for the bone

PREPARATION INSTRUCTIONS

1) Crush walnuts in food processor; set aside in large bowl.

2) Crush carrots in food processor; add to the bowl of walnuts.

3) Place sweet potato, parsley, celery and garlic into food processor; chop until very course. Add mixture to walnuts and carrots, blend well.

4) Blend into mixture lemon juice, grape seed oil, adobo, rosemary, onion powder, nama shoyu, cayenne and salt.

5) Shape patties in the form of a lamb chop, using a thick julienne of Asian pear as the bone. Remove "bone" until later, leaving a groove.

6) Place patties on Teflex sheets and dehydrate for 3½ hours at 150°.

7) Turn patties over; dehydrate for 3½ more hours.

8) Remove to plates; replace "bone" into groove to serve. Serve with spicy mint jelly sauce (see recipe in "Sauce" section).

NOTE:

Adobo seasoning is a dry mixture of sea salt, garlic, onion, black pepper, oregano, bay leaf and turmeric. It comes organically pre-blended, found in the spice section, or you could make your own using the ingredients as listed: largest amount to least.

Marrakesh Open Market Melange (Timbale of Green and Purple Baby Japanese Eggplant)

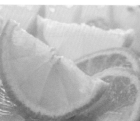

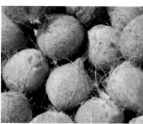

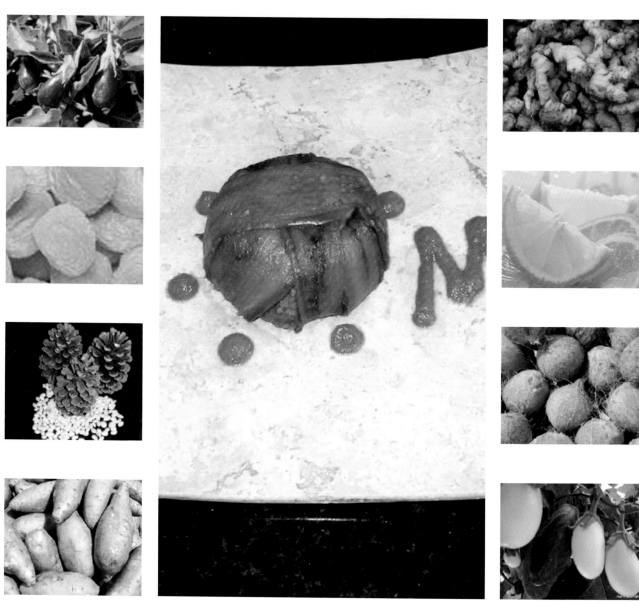

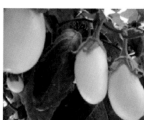

INGREDIENTS

2 green baby Japanese
eggplants

2 purple baby Japanese
eggplants

1 tbsp pine nuts

2 tbsp sweet potato, diced

8 dried apricots

1 tsp lemon zest

1 tsp lemon juice,
fresh squeezed

1 tbsp coconut butter

2 tsp ginger, grated

¼ tsp nutmeg, grated

¼ tsp cinnamon powder

¼ tsp Himalayan sea salt,
for mixture

~~ grape seed oil, for roasting

PREPARATION INSTRUCTIONS

1) Remove outer skin from eggplant; slice lengthwise as thinly as possible on a mandoline. (The purple skinned egg-plant will have darker pulp; the green will have lighter pulp.) Salt lightly and let sit for 1 hour; rinse eggplant under cold water to remove salt. Dry between paper towels; place in bowl.

2) Flavor eggplant slices with grape seed oil, garlic powder and salt. Place on Teflex sheet and dehydrate at 110° for about 2 hours, until soft.

3) Lightly oil the sweet potato. Soak pine nuts in cold water for 1 hour; drain and dry. Place sweet potato and pine nuts on Teflex sheets and dehydrate – sweet potato for 2 hours, pine nuts for 1 hour – at 110°.

4) Soak apricots in cold water until soft; dry well; dice. Place apricots into food processor; add remainder of ingredients. Chop until well blended.

5) Cover inside of 2 ramekins with plastic wrap; drape excess wrap outside. Place eggplant slices into ramekins in a crisscross pattern, alternating green and purple eggplant strips. Slices will overhang ramekins at each end.

6) Fill cavity with vegetable mixture; cover and close with overhanging eggplant slices. Fold draped plastic over the top and press down so that ingredients are tightly packed. Refrigerate if not going to enjoy immediately.

TO SERVE:

Unfold wrap from top of timbale; turn ramekin upside down and remove wrap that was inside ramekin, covering bottom of timbale. Reheat in dehydrator at 105° for 20 minutes; if refrigerated, reheat for 1 hour. Drizzle with roasted red pepper sauce.

Moroccan Sun Kebabs with Roasted Vegetables

INGREDIENTS

8 ounces walnuts, washed and dried

8 ounces carrots, peeled and diced

½ cup sweet potato, peeled, diced

1 tsp nama shoyu

1 tsp garlic powder

3 ounces red pepper

1 tbsp extra virgin olive oil

2 tbsp barbecue sauce

1½ tsp Himalayan sea salt

vegetables of choice

PREPARATION INSTRUCTIONS

1) Crush walnuts in food processor; place in bowl and set aside.

2) Place carrots, sweet potato, red pepper and garlic powder into food processor; crush. Add to bowl of walnuts.

3) Place all ingredients in food processor and add nama shoyu, oil, barbecue sauce and salt. Blend well.

4) Hand form 1¼ inch square patties; place on Teflex sheet and dehydrate for 4 hours at 110° for 4 hours.

5) Gently flip patties over and dehydrate for an additional 3 hours.

6) Skewer patties with alternating roasted (dehydrated) vegetables of your choice.

7) Place filled skewers back into dehydrator for 10 minutes.

8) Remove; decorate with barbecue sauce. Scatter with Incan berries (can be rehydrated by soaking in water).

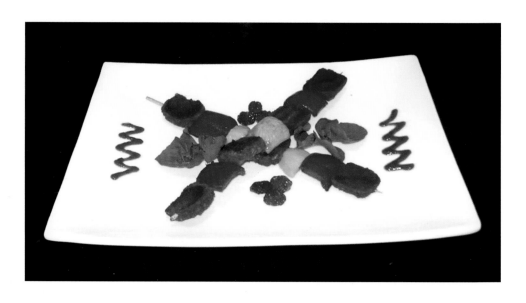

Pad Thai Pasta of Zucchini

INGREDIENTS

2 medium sized green zucchinis

1 tbsp white miso

1 tbsp fresh lime juice

1 tbsp fresh peeled garlic

½ tbsp nama shoyu

1 tbsp sesame seed oil

1 tbsp coconut oil

6 ounces coconut milk

1 tbsp ginger, peeled, diced

2 tbsp almond butter

~~ sea salt to taste

~~ cayenne pepper to taste

~~pomegranate seeds, for garnish

PREPARATION INSTRUCTIONS

1) Cut zucchini, in thin julienne. It can be done with a mandoline or potato peeler (spirooli slicer is excellent.)

2) Spread zucchini on dehydrator tray and dehydrate at 105° for about 30 minutes.

3) For sauce, put all the ingredients (except zucchini) into the blender and blend until smooth. If consistency is too thick, dilute with cold water.

4) Put zucchini in a large bowl and mix with the sauce.

5) Top with grated coconut and chopped cilantro. Garnish with fresh pomegranate seeds.

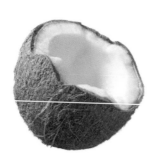
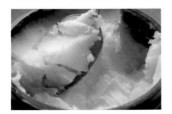
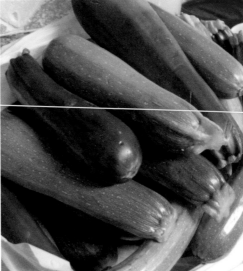
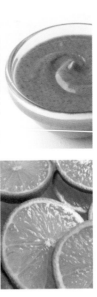

Pasta Basics: Angel Hair, Spaghetti, Fettuccine, Pappardelle

INGREDIENTS

zucchini

summer squash

pattypan squash

acorn squash

cucumber

apple

OIL

extra virgin olive

grape seed

Salba

red palm

garlic powder

onion powder

Himalayan sea salt

PREPARATION INSTRUCTIONS

String pastas are prepared from the same basic recipe; it is the size of the strand that gives each type of pasta its distinctive look. These pastas range in shape from the very small, round angel hair to the large, flat, broad pappardelle.

For our purposes, we will use vegetables to make the pastas. Take any kind of squash, cucumber or apple (for dessert pastas or coleslaws) – whatever you enjoy or fits your recipe – and cut it to the specified shape. You can do this using a knife or a mandoline; you can even use a carrot peeler. I have found that a spiral turning slicer is the best tool for angel hair and spaghetti shapes, while the other tools work better on the thinner, broader shapes.

1) Prepare your vegetable pasta strips accordingly.

2) Coat lightly in the oil of your choice, along with garlic powder, onion powder and sea salt.

3) Spread out loosely on Teflex sheet; dehydrate for 30 minutes at 105°.

4) Mix with the sauce of your choice, following the recipe directions.

Pasta Primo "Bella Serra"

INGREDIENTS

2 zucchinis cut with spiral

½ red bell pepper, seeds removed, cut into julienne strips

1 carrot, peeled, cut with spiral

1 apple, skin on, cut with spiral

1 large jicama, peeled, cut with spiral

1 small beet, cut into fine julienne strips

1½ cup coconut water

3 tbsp apple cider vinegar

2 tbsp nama shoyu

4 tbsp almond butter

1 tbsp turmeric powder

1 tsp garlic powder

4 dates, soaked till soft

1 tsp sea salt

1 cup olive oil

½ cup Zante currants, soaked, dried

PREPARATION INSTRUCTIONS

1) Put in blender: coconut water, apple cider, nama shoyu .

2) Add all other ingredients except olive oil and currants.

3) Blend until smooth.

4) Add olive oil and blend for a few seconds.

5) Mix well with vegetables.

6) Add sea salt to taste.

7) Garnish with Zante currants.

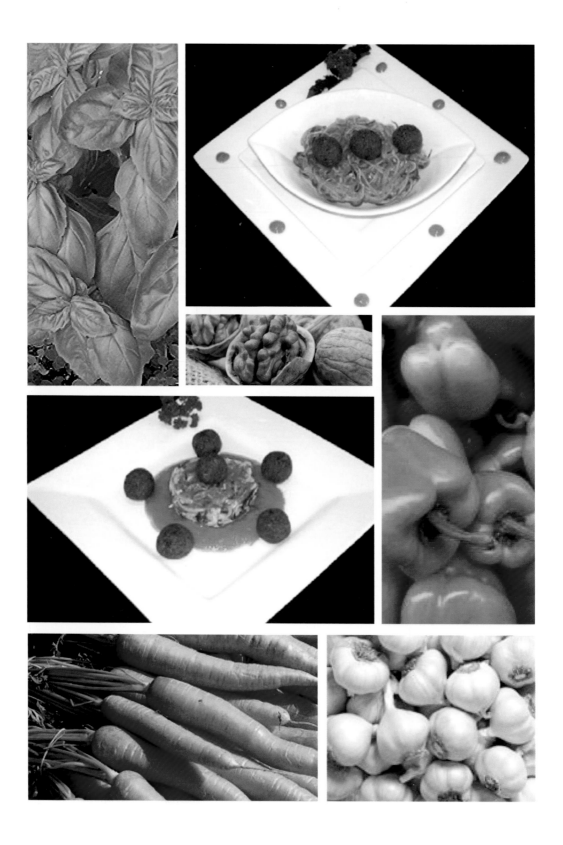

Pattypan Angel Hair with Heaven Drops and Roasted Red Pepper Sauce

INGREDIENTS

HEAVEN DROPS (ITALIAN MEATBALLS)

½ cup walnuts, soaked for 1 hour, well washed and dried

2 ounces raisins, soaked for 20 minutes and dried

2 tsp fresh garlic, peeled, diced

2 ounces carrots, peeled, large diced

½ tsp nama shoyu

1 tbsp red palm oil

1 tsp Himalayan sea salt

1 tsp dried basil

1½ tsp dried Italian herbs

⅛ tsp dried red pepper flakes

1 tbsp ground Salba seeds

1 tsp onion powder

PATTYPAN ANGEL HAIR

3-4 pattypan squash

~~ extra virgin olive oil

~~ garlic powder

~~ onion powder

~~ sea salt

ROASTED RED PEPPER SAUCE

3 red peppers

½ cup red palm oil

1 tbsp garlic powder

1 tbsp onion powder

~~ cayenne

~~ sea salt to taste

PREPARATION INSTRUCTIONS

HEAVEN DROPS

1) Put all ingredients in food processor (except Salba seeds and oil); chop till well mixed.

2) Slowly blend in oil; add Salba seeds and blend all together well.

3) Roll into small balls and place on Teflex sheet. Dehydrate at 110° for 13 hours, turning after 6 hours.

PATTYPAN ANGEL HAIR

1) Cut pattypan squash into thin julienne strips; works best with a spiral turning slicer.

2) Lightly coat strips in oil, salt, garlic and onion powders.

3) Dehydrate on Teflex sheet at 105° for 30 minutes.

RED PEPPER SAUCE

1) Follow directions on the separate red pepper sauce recipe.

TO FINISH

1) Mix sauce and angel hair together, or place angel hair in center of plate, surrounded by sauce. Place heaven drops on and around angel hair.

2) Garnish with sprig of fresh basil.

"Rawsage" Pizza

INGREDIENTS

1 cup walnuts

1 cup water

1 tsp fennel seeds

1 tsp mustard seeds

1 tsp garlic powder

1 tsp onion powder

2 tsp paprika powder

2 tsp nutritional yeast

1 tsp lemon juice

~ sea salt to taste

PREPARATION INSTRUCTIONS

1. Soak walnuts overnight. Rinse very clean; dry between towels. Put walnuts and water into mixer and blend on high speed until well mixed.

2. Put mixture into a cheese cloth and place into a strainer. Close cheese cloth tightly and place a weight on top. Allow mixture to sit at room temperature for 14 hours. Remove and place in bowl – mixture will look like cream cheese.

3. Soak mustard and fennel seeds in lukewarm water for 30 minutes. Drain, dry and blend into walnut cheese mixture. Add remaining ingredients and mix well.

4. Place mixture into the middle of a large sheet of plastic wrap (containing no polyvinyl chloride – best for low temperature dehydrating) and make a cylindrical roll...cigar shaped.

5. Tighten roll by tying one end of the plastic wrap, grasping the other end, and pushing the mixture down toward the tied end. This will condense the mixture and eliminate air pockets. Close and tie the open end and place in freezer for about 4 hours, until mixture is firm.

6. Remove from wrap and cut into very thin slices. Put slices on Teflex sheet and dehydrate at 115° for about 5 hours, flipping slices over about midway. Dehydrate until slices are firm.

7. Construct and assemble pizza by using recipes for Herbed Salba Pizza Crust, Moo-less Macadamia Cheese, and your choice of vegetables. Arrange to your liking with the "rawsage".

Roasted Red Peppers Stuffed with Cilantro Curry Hummus and Ponzu Ginger Dipping Sauce

INGREDIENTS

ROASTED RED PEPPERS

1 red pepper per person

~ extra virgin olive oil for coating

~ sea salt for flavor

CILANTRO CURRY HUMMUS

1 cup sesame seeds (soaked 1 hour and dried)

1 cup pine nuts (soaked 1 hour and dried)

2 tbsp extra virgin olive oil

2 tbsp cold water

1 tbsp nama shoyu

½ tbsp agave

2 tbsp fresh lemon juice

2 tbsp chopped cilantro

1½ tbsp garlic powder

1 tbsp curry powder

1 tsp nutritional yeast

1 tsp Herbamare

~ salt and cayenne to taste

PONZU GINGER DIPPING SAUCE

1 tbsp ponzu

¼ cup nama shoyu

1 tsp grated ginger, liquid removed

1 tsp coconut vinegar

handful nasturtium leaves per plate

PREPARATION INSTRUCTIONS

ROASTED RED PEPPERS

1) Wash and rinse peppers, cut in four equal parts, remove seeds.

2) Flavor with extra virgin olive oil and sea salt.

3) Dehydrate for 6 hours on Teflex sheet (you will have some liquid left; add to hummus).

4) Stuff peppers with hummus and dehydrate about 40 minutes at 110°, until warm.

CILANTRO CURRY HUMMUS

1) Crush sesame seeds and pine nuts in blender; continue blending until smooth.

2) Add all other ingredients except olive oil and cilantro. Slowly add oil when mixture is well blended.

3) Put mixture in bowl and add chopped cilantro. Flavor with salt and cayenne. Spoon onto roasted red peppers.

PONZU GINGER DIPPING SAUCE

1) Blend together the ponzu dipping sauce ingredients and pour into small, individual bowls.

Place bowls of dipping sauce in middle of plates; arrange nasturtium leaves on top of plates. Place hummus-stuffed peppers on top of leaves.

Roasted Vegetable Potpourri

INGREDIENTS

equal amounts of
each vegetable:

red bell pepper

red onion

yellow squash

green zucchini

eggplant

asparagus

herbs and spices to taste

grape seed oil

fresh basil leaves,
fine chopped

fresh rosemary, fine chopped

garlic powder

Herbamare salt

sea salt

PREPARATION INSTRUCTIONS

1) Peel eggplant and cut into ⅛-inch thick lengthwise slices. Using a round cookie cutter (size of cutter to your liking), cut as many round pieces out of the slices as you can get. (You could also cut them into squares with a knife if you prefer.)

2) Toss eggplant with salt (to remove excess water) and let drain for one hour. Refresh eggplant under cold water (also to remove excess salt) and dry between paper towels. Place into a bowl and flavor with grape seed oil and Herbamare. Trim the asparagus and flavor in the same manner. Place both onto Teflex sheets and dehydrate at 105° for about 3 hours, until pliable.

3) Remove seeds from red bell pepper; cut into medium dice. Remove skin from onion; cut into medium size chunks. Cut squash and zucchini into medium dice.

4) Mix the squash, zucchini, onion and red bell pepper together. Flavor with garlic powder, Herbamare and sea salt; add chopped rosemary, basil and grape seed oil. Toss together well.

5) Place on Teflex sheets and dehydrate for about 3½ hours until roasted but still al dente, or to your liking. Toss with herb miso vinaigrette.

6) To serve, place eggplant rounds on dish, top with vegetable potpourri and garnish with asparagus spears.

Root Vegetable Pine Nut Whip

INGREDIENTS

1 cup turnip root,
peeled and cubed

2 cups parsnip,
peeled and cubed

½ cups pine nuts

2 cloves garlic, minced

1 ½ cups water

⅓ cup lemon juice

1 tbsp avocado oil

1½ tsp sea salt

PREPARATION INSTRUCTIONS

1) Put all ingredients into blender and blend until creamy, with a whipped potato-like texture.

2) Finish with snipped chives on top.

Savory Crepe Roll-Up with Vegetables and Wasabi Horseradish Sauce

INGREDIENTS

¾ cup almond flour

¼ cup Salba seeds, ground

¼ cup diced green apple
with skin

¼ cup shredded coconut

1 tbsp maple syrup

1 tbsp Salba oil

½ tsp lemon juice

1 tbsp of coconut oil

½ tsp garlic powder

½ tsp onion powder

½ tsp Himalayan sea salt

½ tsp cinnamon powder

½ tsp fresh chopped thyme

¾ cup water

PREPARATION INSTRUCTIONS

1) Place all ingredients, except Salba seeds, in blender and process on high speed until well blended.

2) Put mixture in bowl, and with a spatula, mix in Salba seeds until well blended.

3) Place in refrigerator for 30 minutes.

4) Spread thinly into 6-inch rounds on dehydrator teflex sheets.

5) Dehydrate for 2 to 3 hour, or until dry but very pliable.

6) Place crepe on plate; spread with small amount of wasabi horseradish sauce. Lay your choice of vegetables (raw or roasted) on one side; roll crepe into tube shape. Cut in half; place one half leaning up against the other.

7) Spoon or squeeze extra sauce over roll-up.

Spaghetti of Zucchini with Nutty Pesto Emulsion

INGREDIENTS

2 medium sized green zucchinis

2 ounces almonds, 2 ounces walnuts, 2 ounces pecans – all soaked 2 hours, well washed, and dried

¼ cup fresh basil, chopped

½ cup fresh parsley, chopped

½ tbsp nama shoyu

~ raisins, soaked 3 hours and dried, for garnish

~ pine nuts, for garnish

1 tbsp white miso

1 juice of one fresh lime

1 tbsp fresh garlic, peeled, large diced

1 cup extra virgin olive oil

1 tbsp ginger peeled, large diced

½ tbsp almond butter

~ water for diluting consistency

~~ sea salt to taste

PREPARATION INSTRUCTIONS

1) Cut zucchini into thin julienne. It can be done with a mandoline or potato peeler (spirooli slicer is excellent.)

2) Spread zucchini on dehydrator tray and dehydrate at 105° for about 20 minutes; set aside.

3) Place almonds, walnuts and pecans in food processor and pulse until course; use spatula to scrape nuts from side of processor and mix together.

4) Add ginger, garlic, almond butter, nama shoyu and miso to nut mixture; pulse until well blended.

5) Add in basil, parsley and oils to mixture, pulse and mix all ingredients together very well. Dilute with water and lime juice to desired consistency.

6) Put zucchini in a large bowl and mix with the sauce.

7) Garnish each individual plate with pine nuts and raisins.

Stuffed Roasted Peppers with Cilantro Curry Hummus and Herb Vinaigrette

INGREDIENTS

4 red peppers

~~ grape seed oil

~~ salt and pepper

HUMMUS

2 cups sesame seeds, soaked 1 hour

2 cups pine nuts, soaked 6 hours

3 tbsp grape seed oil

¼ cup water

1 tbsp agave

½ tsp Himalayan sea salt

1 tsp Herbamare (herb salt)

2 tbsp fresh lemon juice

1 tbsp nama shoyu

2 tbsp fresh cilantro, chopped

1 tsp nutritional yeast

1 tsp garlic powder

1 tbsp curry powder

~~ cayenne to taste

PREPARATION INSTRUCTIONS

RED PEPPERS

1) Wash outside and remove tops of peppers; clean out seeds and pith. Keep bottom intact.

2) Brush with grape seed oil and flavor with salt and pepper.

3) Dehydrate at 105° for about 12 hours or until peppers look roasted; set aside.

HUMMUS

1) Place all ingredients (except for cilantro) in the blender and blend on high speed until all ingredients are well blended. Add cilantro to mixture after main ingredients are blended. If mixture is too thick, it can be diluted by adding water.

TO FINISH

1) One half hour before serving, reheat peppers in dehydrator and stuff with hummus.

• Serve with herb vinaigrette dressing.

• Place peppers in the middle of the plate and garnish with vinaigrette.

• Serve with diced kalamata olives around vinaigrette.

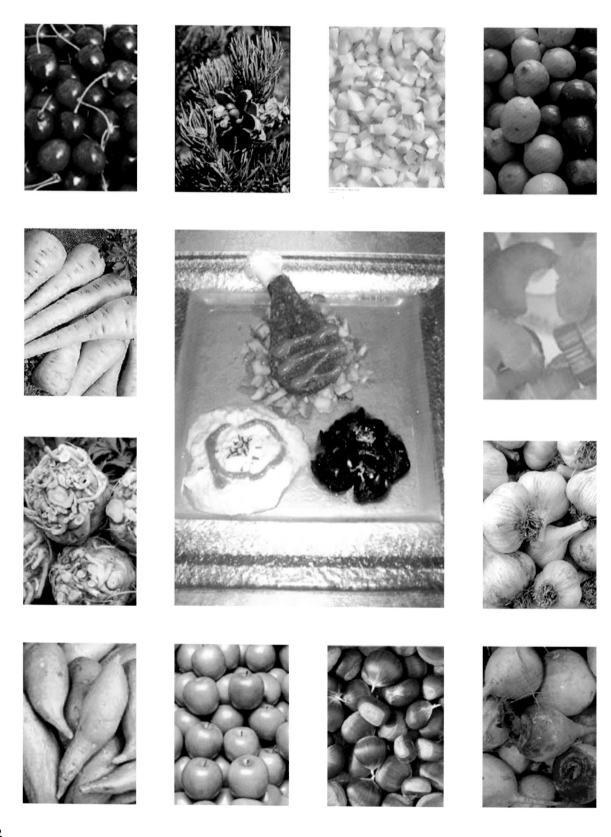

Turkey Leggings

INGREDIENTS

1 cup hanna white sweet potato, peeled, small diced

¼ cup celery root, peeled, small diced

¼ cup Honey Crisp apple, peeled, cored, diced

¼ cup soft chestnuts, clean-prepped*

¼ cup pine nuts

¼ cup onion, peeled diced

2 tbsp grape seed oil

¾ tsp sea salt

½ tsp Bell's seasoning

PREPARATION INSTRUCTIONS

1) Soak pine nuts for 1 hour and drain.

2) Place chestnuts on Teflex sheet and dehydrate at 105° until soft. Do not over-dehydrate, as chestnuts will become hard.

3) Flavor celery root with small amount of grape seed oil and sea salt. Place on Teflex sheet and dehydrate at 105° until soft.

4) Put celery root into food processor and chop until it is a very fine grind.

5) Add remaining ingredients, except grape seed oil, into food processor and chop finely. Slowly drizzle oil into mixture.

6) Shape small patties into the form of a turkey drumstick; place on Teflex sheet and dehydrate for 13 hours at 110°, turning after 6 hours.

Note: *To clean-prep chestnuts, thoroughly wash and dry; remove any dark skins.

Young Coconut Pad Thai with Almond Chili Sauce

INGREDIENTS

4 tbsp xylitol

1 tbsp nama shoyu

1 tsp tamarind

1 tbsp minced garlic

1 tbsp jalapeño, minced

1 tbsp extra virgin olive oil

¼ tsp Himalaya sea salt

1 cup julienne zucchini

1 cup finely shredded
red cabbage

½ cup julienne red onions

1 cup julienne carrots

1 cup julienne Granny Smith
apple, skin on

½ cup julienne red pepper

2 tbsp cilantro leaves

2 cups young Thai
coconut meat

salt and pepper to taste

ALMOND CHILI SAUCE

½ cup raw almond butter

1 tbsp minced, peeled
fresh ginger

1 Thai chili pepper or jalapeño

2 tbsp fresh lemon juice

4 tbsp xylitol

1 tbsp nama shoyu

½ cup of water, if needed,
to thin

salt and pepper to taste

PREPARATION INSTRUCTIONS

PAD THAI

1) In blender, on high speed, combine xylitol, nama shoyu, garlic, jalapeño, oil, tamarind and salt. Process until smooth.

2) Place zucchini, red cabbage, carrots, onion, apples, red bell peppers, coconut meat and cilantro in a bowl; mix the vegetables with the oil mixture (from step 1).

ALMOND CHILI SAUCE

1) In the blender, add all ingredients and blend until smooth, adding water to thin if necessary. The sauce should have the consistency of melted ice cream. Season to taste with salt and pepper.

TO FINISH

1) Arrange the pad Thai mixture in the center of the plate.

2) Spoon some almond chili sauce on the top of the pad thai; garnish plate with the rest of the chili sauce.

3) Decorate with toasted pecan and raisins.

Zucchini Fettuccine Alfredo with Peas and a Heart-Beet

INGREDIENTS

2 medium sized green zucchinis

½ cup peas (can use frozen, thawed)

1 tbsp white miso

1 tbsp apple cider vinegar

1 tbsp fresh peeled garlic

½ tbsp worcestershire sauce

1 tbsp grape seed oil

¾ cup almond milk

1 tbsp ginger, peeled, diced

2 tbsp almond butter

~~ Herbamare salt to taste

~~ cayenne pepper to taste

~~ Italian parsley, chopped, for garnish

~~ beets, thinly sliced**

PREPARATION INSTRUCTIONS

1) Cut zucchini in thin julienne. It can be done with a mandoline or potato peeler (spirooli slicer is excellent.)

2) Spread zucchini on dehydrator tray and dehydrate at 105° for about 30 minutes.

3) For sauce, put all the ingredients (except zucchini, peas and parsley) into the blender and blend until smooth. If consistency is too thick, dilute with cold water.

4) Put zucchini and peas in a large bowl and combine with the sauce.

5) Top with heart-beet; garnish with chopped Italian parsley.

**Slice beets into thin rounds; flavor and dehydrate for 30 minutes. Remove and cut into heart shape with cookie cutter.

Beverages

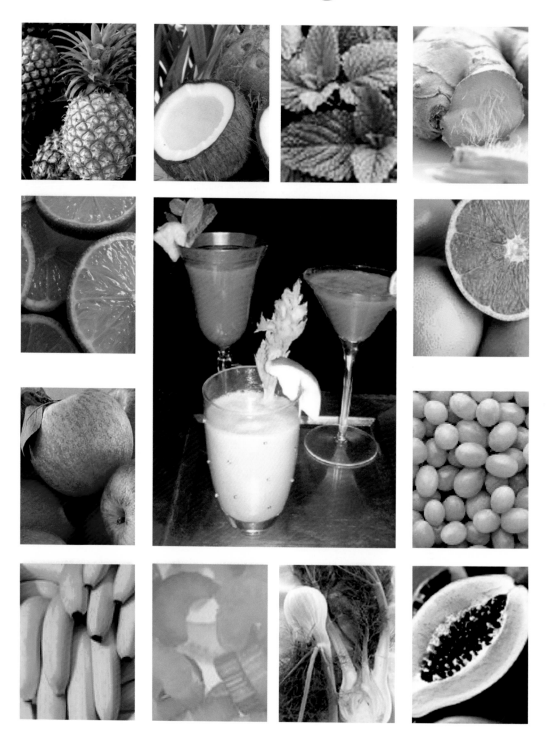

Almond Milk

INGREDIENTS

3 cups raw almonds

6 cups water

¼ tsp nutmeg

1 tbsp vanilla extract

¼ tsp cinnamon

PREPARATION INSTRUCTIONS

1. Place 3 cups of raw almonds in water. Soak for 12 hours. Drain water and rinse.

2. Blend almonds with water.

3. Double strain mixture through a cheesecloth or coffee filter. Add nutmeg, cinnamon, and vanilla extract to mixture. (Save and store almond pulp for use in making almond flour – see "Bites" section).

4. Store in an airtight container in the refrigerator for up to 3 days.

NOTE:

If time is limited, you can buy good organic almond milk in most health food stores.

Apple Almond Wake-Me-Up

INGREDIENTS

2 cups almond milk

8 ounces almonds, soaked, washed, dried

1 avocado, ripe, large chopped

6 ounces Fuji apple, peeled, cored, chopped

1 tbsp maca

1 tbsp white agave

1 tbsp extra virgin coconut oil

1 tsp cinnamon powder

1 tsp cayenne

1 cup ice

PREPARATION INSTRUCTIONS

1) Place all ingredients in blender.

2) Blend at high speed until fully mixed.

NOTE

This is a great wake up drink to get your day started.

Coconut Milk

INGREDIENTS

basic coconut milk

4½ cups water, warm or room temperature

2 cups shredded dried coconut

pinch of salt

SEE BELOW FOR ALTERNATE FLAVORS

agave, combined with:

vanilla

chocolate

carob

citrus

PREPARATION INSTRUCTIONS

BASIC COCONUT MILK

1) Soak the coconut – covered – in the water for about 30 minutes.

2) Transfer to a blender and blend until smooth.

3) Strain through a strainer lined with a cheesecloth.

FOR ALTERNATE FLAVORS,

Add the Following to the Basic Coconut Milk

- Vanilla, add 2 tsp vanilla extract and 2 tsp of agave.

- Chocolate or carob, add 2 tsp of your preferred flavor-powder and 2 tsp of agave.

- Citrus (orange, lemon or lime work equally well), add 2 tsp of fresh juice and 2 tsp of agave.

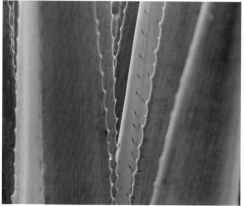

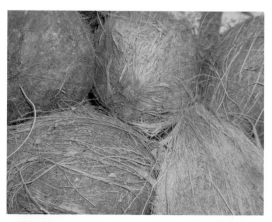

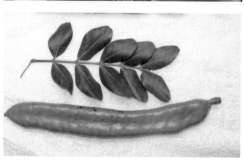

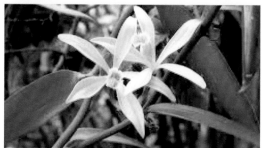

Dandy Green Delight

INGREDIENTS

5 celery stalks, washed and dried

5 kale leaves, with stems intact, washed and dried

5 dandelion leaves, with stems intact, washed and dried

1 tbsp maca

3 Fuji or Gala apples, skin on, cored and cut into eight slices

1 tsp fresh peeled ginger

1 tsp fresh peeled garlic

~~ cayenne to taste

PREPARATION INSTRUCTIONS

1) Place all ingredients – except maca --through a heavy-duty juicer, obtaining a nutritious blended drink.

2) Stir maca into mixture before drinking.

Note:

The recipe can be varied by replacing the celery, kale or dandelions with 2 small beets, peeled and chopped.

Fennel, Grapefruit, Celery and Apple Juice

INGREDIENTS

3 cups fennel, well cleaned

2 celery stalks, well cleaned

1 Fuji apple

1 cup freshly squeezed grapefruit juice

PREPARATION INSTRUCTIONS

1) Clean and chop fennel.

2) Clean and chop celery.

3) Leave skin on apple; core and cut into eight slices.

4) Put celery, fennel and apple through a heavy-duty juicer; stir in grapefruit juice.

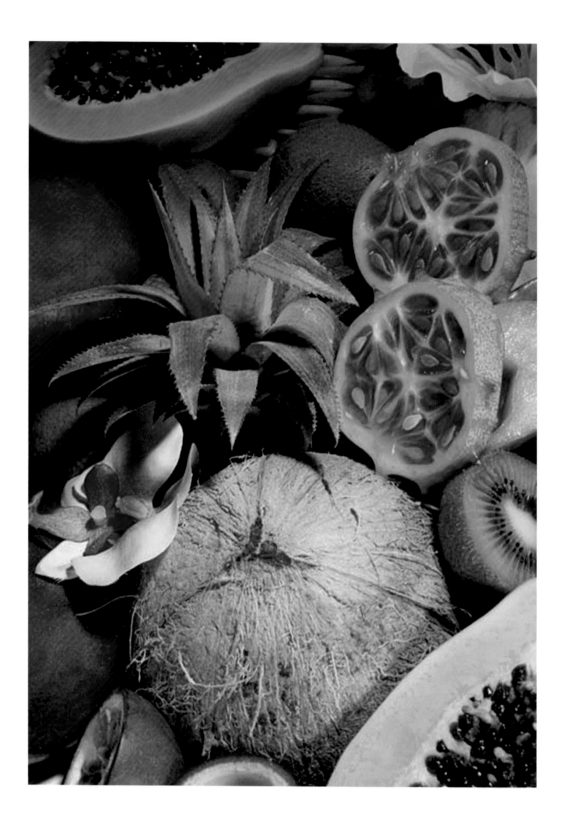

Green Smoothies

INGREDIENTS

1 bunch arugula

4 Gala apples

½ lime with peel

½ banana, peeled

2 cups water

1 tsp ground cinnamon

16 frozen white grapes

1 tsp of raw ginger, peeled

⅛ tsp cayenne pepper

PREPARATION INSTRUCTIONS

1) Place all ingredients in blender.

2) Blend on high speed until thoroughly mixed and obtaining desired consistency.

3) Dilute with more water if necessary.

Sunny Island Aperitif

INGREDIENTS

2 cups ripe papaya, cubed

2 cups ripe pineapple, cubed

30 mint leaves

8 ounces coconut water

1 tbsp agave

1 tbsp lime juice, fresh squeezed

1 tbsp ginger juice, fresh squeezed

PREPARATION INSTRUCTIONS

1) Place all ingredients in blender.

2) Blend at high speed until fully mixed.

3) Serve with slice of lime on rim of glass.

Bites

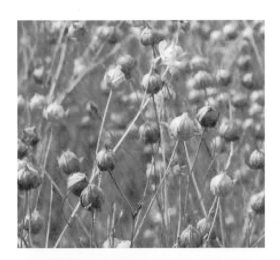
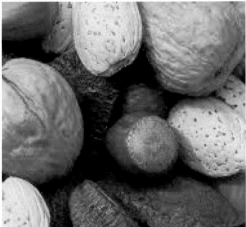
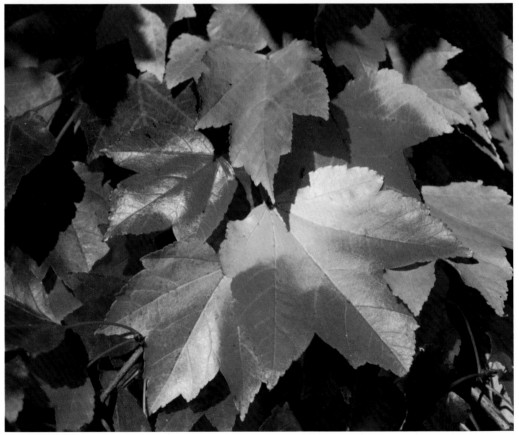

Almond Brittle Crunch

INGREDIENTS

½ cup coarsely ground almonds

soak and dry almonds; place in Cuisinart and coarsely grind to yield ½ cup

½ tsp almond extract

½ cup maple syrup

¼ cup flax meal

~~ Himalayan sea salt

PREPARATION INSTRUCTIONS

1) Pull all ingredients in food processor and blend until well mixed.

2) Spread very thin on a Teflex sheet and dehydrate at 105° for 12 hours.

3) Remove from Teflex sheet and flip over onto a screen and dehydrate for another 24 hours.

4) Cut into strips or break into large chunks.

Almond Flour

INGREDIENTS

3 cups raw almonds

6 cups water

PREPARATION INSTRUCTIONS

1) Place 3 cups of raw almonds in water. Soak for 12 hours. Drain water and rinse.

2) Blend almonds with water. Double strain mixture through a cheesecloth or coffee filter.

3) Using an offset spatula, spread the pulp on Teflex sheet, place on a dehydrator shelf.

4) Dehydrate at 105° for 24 hours or until completely dry.

5) Transfer the dehydrated pulp to a food processor and grind it to a silky flour.

NOTE:

Save for future plain almond milk use in recipes, or add ¼ tsp each of nutmeg and cinnamon with 1 tbsp vanilla extract for drinking. See "Beverage" section. Milk can be stored in an airtight container in the refrigerator for up to 3 days.

Candied Pecans

INGREDIENTS

2 cups raw pecan halves, soaked in water 6 hours, drained and dried

2 tbsp maple syrup

1 tbsp cinnamon powder

1 tsp ginger powder

1 tsp Himalayan sea salt

PREPARATION INSTRUCTIONS

1) Place pecans in a bowl, add the maple syrup, ginger, cinnamon powder and sea salt. Toss to coat.

2) Spread the pecan halves on a Teflex sheet.

3) Dehydrate at 105° for 24 hours or until crisp.

Cinnamon Walnuts

INGREDIENTS

2 cups raw walnuts, soaked in water for 8 hours, drained and dried

¼ tsp garam masala

1 tbsp ground cinnamon

1 tsp cumin powder

2 tbsp maple syrup

touch cayenne

¼ tsp sea salt

PREPARATION INSTRUCTIONS

1) Place the walnuts in a bowl, adding the maple syrup, cayenne, garam masala, cinnamon and sea salt. Mix well to coat walnuts.

2) Spread walnuts on a Teflex sheet.

3) Dehydrate at 105° for 20 hours or until crisp. Turn walnuts over after 12 hours.

Crispy Fruit Chips

INGREDIENTS

FRESH HARD TREE FRUITS*

pears

apples

Asian pears

~~ maple syrup

~~ cinnamon

~~ nutmeg

~~ lemon juice

~~ black pepper, to finish

PREPARATION INSTRUCTIONS

1) Slice fruit very thin on mandoline.

2) Put all other ingredients, except pepper, into bowl; mix. Amount of flavoring ingredients is up to your liking.

3) Toss thinly sliced fruits into flavoring mix.

4) Place fruit slices onto Teflex sheet and dehydrate at 105° until crisp.

5) Finish with a sprinkle of black pepper.

NOTE:

Dehydrating times to achieve crispness vary with the type of fruit. Normally the time is over 16 hours.

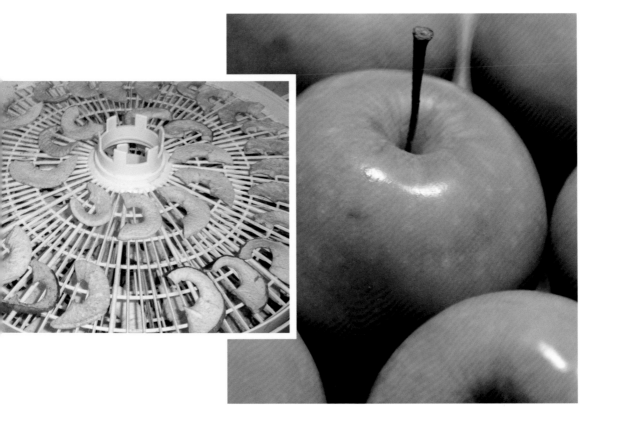

Dragola Crackers

INGREDIENTS

1½ cups golden flax seed

2½ cups water

1 tsp cumin powder

2 tsp maple sugar

1 tsp cinnamon

1½ tsp chili powder

½ tsp cayenne powder

1 tsp minced ginger

½ tsp garam masala

1 tbsp minced red onion

1 tbsp minced fresh garlic

1 tbsp nama shoyu

1 tbsp grape seed oil

1 tbsp sea salt

PREPARATION INSTRUCTIONS

1) Combine flaxseed and water in a bowl and soak for 6 hours or until the seeds absorb all of the water.

2) In a food processor, combine the soaked seeds, and all the ingredients. Add the grape seed oil slowly, at the end when it is a nice mixture (it will look like a bread dough mixture).

3) Spread the flaxseed mixture in a ⅛ inch thick layer on a nonstick drying sheet or Teflex. Place on dehydrator shelves and dehydrate at 105° for about 8 hours or until firm enough to flip the cracker sheets onto the dehydrator shelves.

4) Once the sheets are on the shelves, cut into 2 to 4 inch pieces (pizza cutter is best for this). Continue to dehydrate for about 12 hours more, or until crisp.

Can use immediately, or store in an airtight container at room temperature for up to 2 weeks. This is great instead of bread.

To make cracker crumbs, place the crackers in a heavy duty plastic bag and crush with a rolling pin.

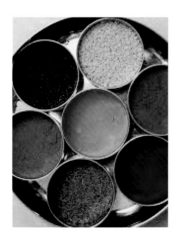
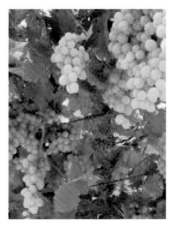
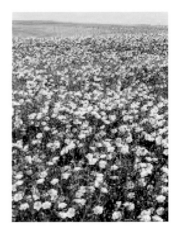

Ginger Pumpkin Seeds

INGREDIENTS

2 cups pumpkin seeds, soaked for 10 hours and drained

2 tbsp freshly squeezed ginger juice **

1 tbsp white raw agave

½ tsp sea salt

1 tsp cumin powder

touch of cayenne

PREPARATION INSTRUCTIONS

1) To get freshly squeezed ginger juice, peel and grate ginger in food processor until very fine. Put ginger in the palm of your hand and squeeze juice over a small bowl. Repeat this until you have enough juice. **

2) In a small bowl, add ginger juice, salt, cumin and cayenne, whisk all together and finish by adding raw white agave. Mix in the pumpkin seeds and let sit for 10 minutes.

3) Place the pumpkin seeds on a Teflex sheet and spread evenly over the sheet.

4) Dehydrate at 105° for about 16 hours. Remove and store in glass jars. Can remain in the glass jars, refrigerated for months. Keep lids tightly closed.

**Or, give yourself a break and buy a jar of squeezed 100% ginger juice at any organic or health food store.

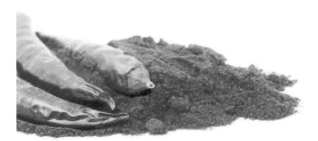

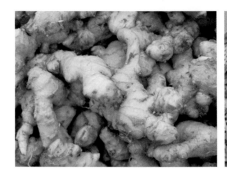

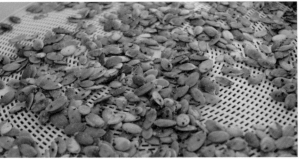

Herb Garlic Onion Crust

INGREDIENTS

1 large yellow onion

¼ cup ground flaxseed

¼ cup sunflower seeds

¼ cup nama shoyu

2 ounces olive oil

1 tsp ground garlic powder

2 tbsp mixture
fresh chopped herbs:
(thyme, rosemary, oregano)

1 tsp sea salt

PREPARATION INSTRUCTIONS

1) Peel and halve the onion; cut into fine slices. Put into a large mixing bowl.

2) Add all remaining ingredients into a food processor; pulse 6 times, using an "S" blade. Scrape sides of the bowl.

3) Spread mixture thinly on a Teflex sheet and dehydrate at 105° for 11 hours. Crust will be pliable.

4) Flip crust and dehydrate for another hour. Cut into squares.

NOTE:

Do not over-dehydrate or crust will dry out and will not be pliable.

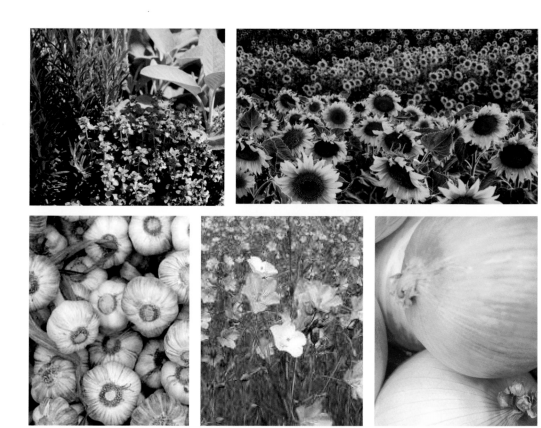

Herbed Salba Pizza Crust

INGREDIENTS

1 large yellow onion

¼ cup Salba seeds (whole)

¼ cup sunflower seeds

¼ cup nama shoyu

2 tbsp and 2 tsp grape seed oil

1 tsp ground garlic

1 tbsp mixture fresh chopped herbs: (thyme, basil, oregano)

½ tsp sea salt

PREPARATION INSTRUCTIONS

1) Peel and halve the onion; slice using slicing blade in food processor; set aside.

2) In a medium sized bowl, add the following in order: nama shoyu, all grape seed oil, garlic and salt. Blend well. Add in Salba whole seeds, sunflower seeds and herbs, making sure they are well coated.

3) Add sliced onions; mix again and let mixture sit for 15 minutes until all ingredients are incorporated well. Put mixture into food processor and pulse 8 times to further grind ingredients.

4) Pour mixture (dough) out of food processor bowl and place on Teflex sheet; smooth out to make a ⅛ inch thick, 13 inch round.

5) Dehydrate at 105° for 7 hours, until it is firm enough to flip on dehydrator shelves. Flip crust and continue dehydrating for about 10 hours until dough is firm and crisp.

Dough can be stored in refrigerator (wrapped in plastic), until it is ready to be finished with sauce, vegetables, other condiments, etc.

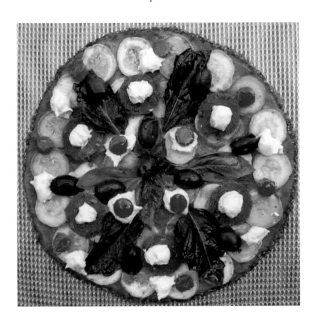

Krunchy, Krispy Kale Kracklins

INGREDIENTS

1 bunch fresh kale

DRESSING

9 ounces sesame tahini

3 ounces nama shoyu

3 ounces apple cider vinegar

3 ounces water

juice of 1 lemon

1½ bunches scallions

1 garlic clove

3 ounces nutritional yeast

1 tbsp cumin powder

~ sea salt to taste

~ white sesame seeds for finished coating

PREPARATION INSTRUCTIONS

1) Wash and dry kale leaves extremely well; remove stems; set aside.

2) Put all dressing ingredients into blender and blend on high speed until completely mixed.

3) Put ⅔ dressing into large bowl (save remaining ⅓ for later use); add kale leaves and coat all the leaves with the dressing to well incorporate each leaf with dressing.

4) Place leaves on Teflex sheets, sprinkle with sea salt; dehydrate at 115° for about 4 hours, until crisp.

5) Pour remainder of dressing into a squeeze bottle. Squeeze this dressing generously over dehydrated kale leaves; sprinkle with white sesame seeds.

6) Continue dehydrating leaves for about another 3 hours, until well crisped.

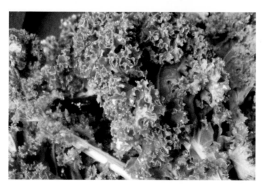

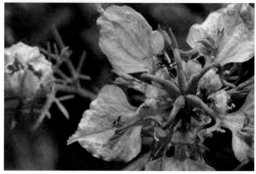

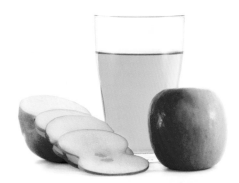

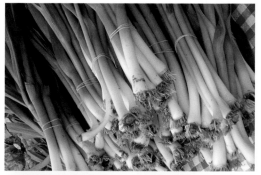

Picante Brazil Nuts

INGREDIENTS

1 cup raw Brazil nuts,
soaked in water for 16 hours,
drained and dried

1 tbsp maple sugar

1½ tsp chili powder

1 tsp ground cayenne pepper

½ tsp Himalayan sea salt

PREPARATION INSTRUCTIONS

1) Place the Brazil nuts in a bowl, adding the maple sugar, chili powder, cayenne, and sea salt. Toss to coat.

2) Spread the Brazil nuts on a nonstick drying sheet.

3) Place sheet on dehydrator shelf and dehydrate at 105° for 28 hours or until crisp.

4) Store nuts in glass jar.

Pickled Ginger

INGREDIENTS

2 tbsp fresh ginger, peeled and finely sliced

¼ cup apple cider vinegar

1 tbsp agave

1 tbsp turmeric

PREPARATION INSTRUCTIONS

1) Place all ingredients in a container with a lid; seal.

2) Shake to combine.

3) Keep in container for 24 hours before using; can store for up to 10 days.

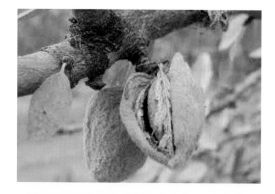

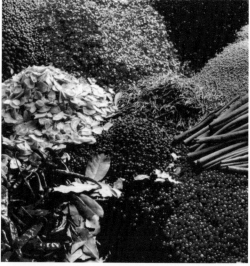

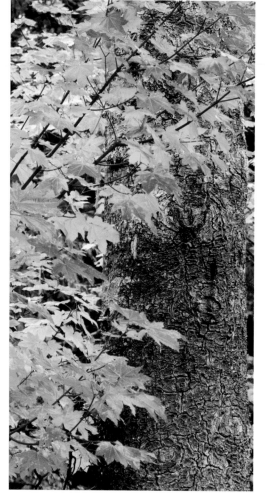

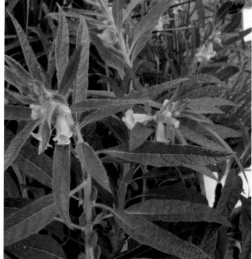

Sesame Brittle Crunch

INGREDIENTS

½ cup sesame seeds

½ cup maple syrup

¼ cup almond flour

½ tsp ground ginger

~~ Himalayan sea salt

PREPARATION INSTRUCTIONS

1) Pull all ingredients in food processor and blend until well mixed.

2) Spread very thin on a Teflex sheet and dehydrate at 105° for 12 hours.

3) Remove from Teflex sheet and flip over onto a screen and dehydrate for another 24 hours.

4) Cut into strips or break into large chunks.

Spicy Caramelized Almonds

INGREDIENTS

2 cups raw almonds, soaked in water for 12 hours, drained and dried

2 tbsp maple syrup

1 tbsp cayenne pepper

1 tbsp ginger powder

1 tbsp cumin powder

1 tbsp Himalayan sea salt

PREPARATION INSTRUCTIONS

1) Place the almonds in a bowl, adding the maple syrup, cayenne, ginger, cumin and sea salt. Toss to coat almonds.

2) Spread the almonds on Teflex sheet.

3) Dehydrate at 105° for 24 hours or until crisp.

Desserts

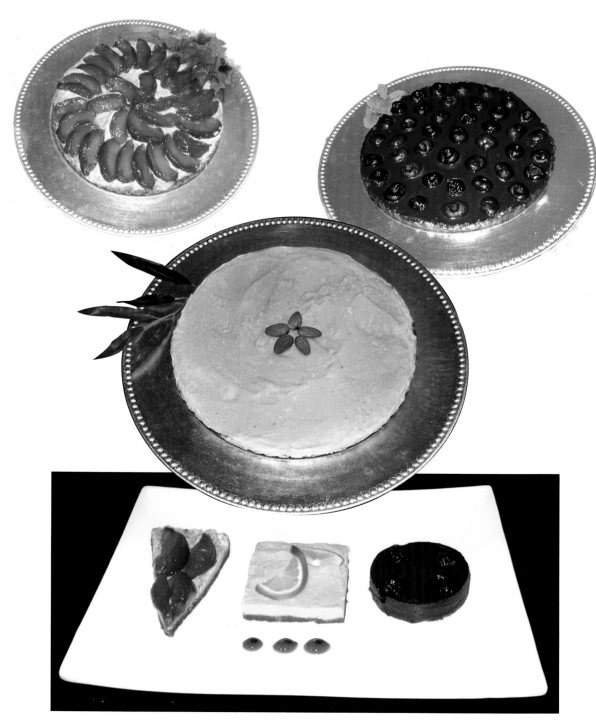

Almond Pomegranate Tapioca

INGREDIENTS

ALMOND POMEGRANATE EMULSION

1 quart almond milk

½ cup pomegranate juice concentrate

1 tbsp lemon juice

TAPIOCA

3 cups almond pomegranate emulsion, slightly warm

½ cup Salba seeds

1 fresh pomegranate, seeds removed

PREPARATION INSTRUCTIONS

1) Put pomegranate juice concentrate, lemon juice and almond milk into blender and blend well. Emulsion will be slightly warm from blender.

2) Immediately place 3 cups of the emulsion and Salba seeds in glass jar with tight fitting lid. Store the remainder of the emulsion refrigerated in a glass jar.

3) Cap and shake jar vigorously for 15 seconds. Let stand for 1 minute and shake again. Place in refrigerator; allow to set up and gel for 30 minutes before using.

4) Place pomegranate seeds into bottom of stemmed glasses. Pour tapioca over seeds to serve; top with a spicy, caramelized almond.

NOTE:

Other concentrates can be used in place of pomegranate, along with diced pieces of the fruit, such as raspberry, peach, cherry, etc.

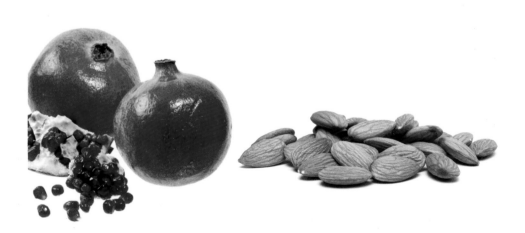

Apple Ginger Citrus Delights

INGREDIENTS

8 ounces Gala or Fuji apples, peeled

3 ounces almonds, soaked and dried

1 tsp fresh ginger, peeled and grated

3 ounces raisins, soaked and dried

1 tbsp lucuma powder

1 ounce cinnamon powder

1 tsp fresh lemon juice

3 tbsp raw agave

PREPARATION INSTRUCTIONS

1) Slice half of the apples (4 ounces) with slicing blade in food processor; place in bowl.

2) Shred remaining half of apples with shredding blade in food processor; add to sliced apples.

3) Fine-grind almonds in bottom of food processor using "S" blade. Add to apple mixture, blend well.

4) Add remaining ingredients and mix well.

5) Press mixture into individual rounds, approximately 1 inch thick.

6) Place onto Teflex sheet and dehydrate for about 5 hours at 105°.

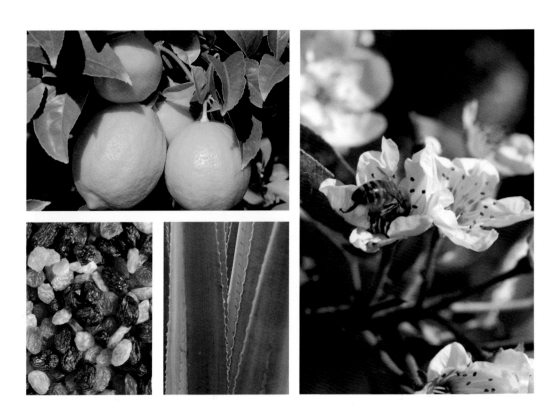

Banana Ice Cream

INGREDIENTS

1 cup homemade almond milk

2 tsp cinnamon powder

½ tsp vanilla extract

chocolate chips or shavings
for garnish

2 fresh bananas, peeled and
cut into 4 pieces

4 frozen, peeled bananas, cut
into large pieces

banana chips for garnish

PREPARATION INSTRUCTIONS

1) Pour almond milk into blender. Add frozen bananas, cinnamon and vanilla extract. Place fresh bananas on top.

2) Process in blender on high speed, using tamper to push down the bananas. This will make the mixture creamy.

3) Continue blending until the mixture forms the look of ice cream.

4) Garnish with banana chips and chocolate chips or shavings.

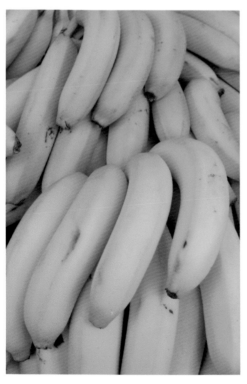

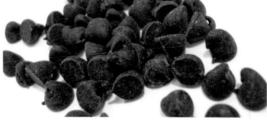

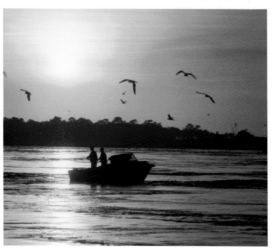

Caramelized Peach Torte with Pecan Date Crust and Almond Cream Filling

INGREDIENTS

9-INCH PECAN DATE CRUST

2 cups pecans, soaked overnight, drained and dried

1 cup pitted dates, soaked for 20 minutes if dry (save water after draining dates; use for smoothies)

½ tsp Himalayan sea salt

1 lemon, grated to a very fine zest

ALMOND CREAM FILLING

1 cup almonds soaked overnight

½ cup coconut meat

1 tbsp maple syrup

⅓ cup coconut butter

1 tbsp almond extract

1 tsp lemon juice

~~ sea salt

CARAMELIZED PEACHES

4 to 5 large peaches, washed**

2 tbsp white agave

1 tbsp lemon juice

PREPARATION INSTRUCTIONS

PECAN DATE CRUST

1) Blend ingredients together in food processor until fine. The mixture will be gooey.

2) Press into a 9-inch pie pan. Place in dehydrator at 110° for 6 hours.

ALMOND CREAM FILLING

1) Pulse almonds and coconut meat together until fine and well blended.

2) Add remaining ingredients to blender and process till mixture is creamy.

3) Cover bottom of crust; refrigerate for 6 hours.

CARAMELIZED PEACHES

1) Cut peaches in half; remove pits; cut each half into 3 slices.

2) Mix together in bowl agave and lemon juice. Place peach slices into bowl, and coat with mixture, being careful not to break the flesh of the peaches.

3) Cover bowl, let peaches sit for ½ hour; remove peaches; drain and place on Teflex sheet. Dehydrate at 110° for 3 hours until peaches are soft and well caramelized.

TO FINISH

1) Decorate top of filling with peach slices. **You may use as many peach slices as you like. If you cannot find large peaches, 6 to 8 small peaches should cover the top to your liking. Refrigerate for 1 hour before serving.

2) Garnish with raspberry sauce and fresh berries.

This torte can also be made substituting plums, apricots and/or nectarines.

Chia Mango Mint Mousse

INGREDIENTS

6 tbsp chia seeds

½ cup coconut milk

½ cup coconut water

1 cup assorted fresh or frozen diced, ripe mangos

3 tbsp xylitol

2 tbsp lemon juice

1 tsp spearmint flavor

fresh mint leaves for garnish

PREPARATION INSTRUCTIONS

1) Soak the chia seeds in the coconut water until they expand or bloom. They will look like small, dark tapioca beads. It can be started before going to bed, so it can be ready in the morning.

2) Add all ingredients into a high-speed blender and blend until smooth.

3) Garnish with fresh mint leaves.

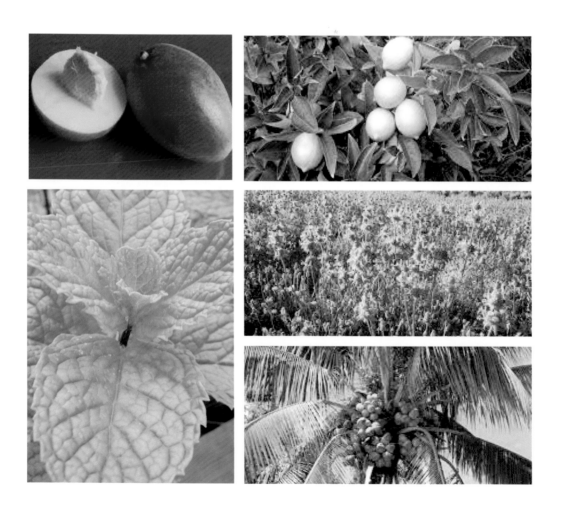

Chilled Berries Chia Parfait

INGREDIENTS

3 tbsp chia seeds

½ cup coconut milk

½ cup coconut water

1 cup assorted fresh or
frozen berries

1 tbsp maple syrup

1 tbsp lemon juice

~~ sea salt

PREPARATION INSTRUCTIONS

1) Soak the chia seeds in the coconut water, until they expand or blossom. They will look like tapioca. It can be started before going to bed, so it can be ready in the morning.

2) Add all ingredients into a high-speed blender and blend until smooth.

3) Alternate layers of parfait with fresh berries in a clear glass.

NOTE:

To get some extra flavor, add a touch of cayenne to the blender at the last minute.

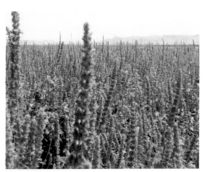

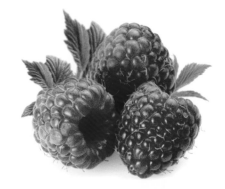

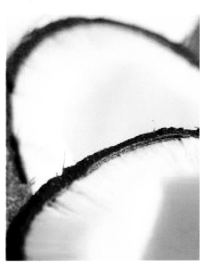

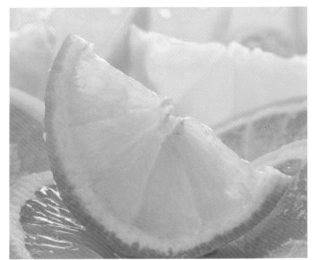

Coconut Macaroons

INGREDIENTS

3 cups shredded, dried coconut

¼ cup raw white agave

1 tbsp maple syrup

1 tsp almond extract

1 tsp coconut extract

1 tsp of vanilla extract

¼ cup coconut oil

½ tsp sea salt

PREPARATION INSTRUCTIONS

1) Put all ingredients into food processor and pulse until ingredients are well mixed. Scrape sides of bowl with spatula during this process to include all of mixture.

2) Put mixture into refrigerator for 15 minutes.

3) Form small balls by hand or use ice cream scoop to form balls.

4) Place on tray and put in dehydrator. Dehydrate at 105° for about 3 hours or until macaroon is crispy outside and soft inside.

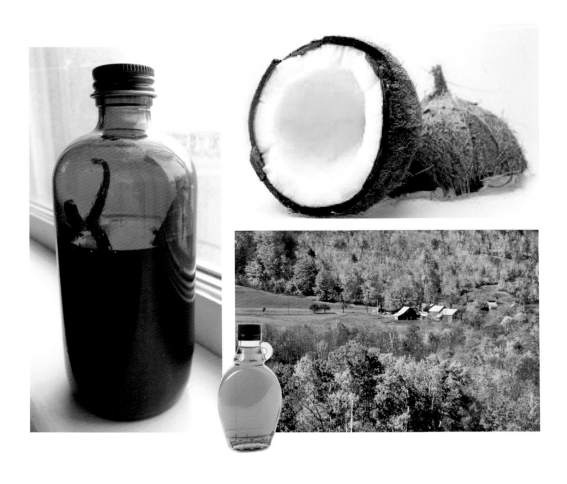

Double Dark Chocolate Pudding

INGREDIENTS

1 cup fresh young Thai coconut meat, cut into small cubes **

¼ cup coconut water

2 ounces prepared Irish moss (per instructions on package)

1 tbsp vanilla powder (or liquid)

¼ cup coconut milk

¼ cup maple syrup

¼ cup raw cocoa powder

2 tbsp mesquite powder

~~ touch of sea salt

PREPARATION INSTRUCTIONS

1) Put all ingredients in blender and puree on high speed until mixture is completely smooth, stopping to scrape the sides as necessary.

2) Serve over fresh berries in a martini glass.

3) Garnish with sesame brittle crunch.

NOTE:

If fresh young Thai coconut meat is not available, use dried, shredded coconut and soak in water for 1 hour prior to using.

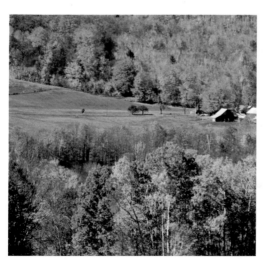
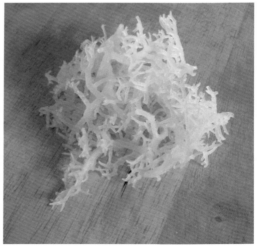

Fudgy Chocolate Torte With Walnut Date Crust and Caramelized Cherries

INGREDIENTS

9-INCH WALNUT DATE CRUST

2 cups walnuts, soaked overnight, drained and dried

1 cup pitted dates, soaked for 20 minutes if dry (save water after straining dates; use for smoothies)

½ tsp Himalayan sea salt

1 lemon, grated to a very fine zest

FUDGY CHOCOLATE FILLING

1 cup cocoa powder

1 cup maple syrup

1 cup coconut butter

1 tsp vanilla extract

CARAMELIZED CHERRIES

30 fresh cherries, pits removed

2 tbsp white agave

1 tbsp lemon juice

PREPARATION INSTRUCTIONS

WALNUT DATE CRUST

1) Blend ingredients together in food processor until fine. The mixture will be gooey.

2) Press into a 9-inch pie pan. Place in dehydrator at 110° for 6 hours.

FUDGY CHOCOLATE FILLING

1) Blend all of the filling ingredients in a blender on high speed until smooth. Pour into the torte crust.

2) Decorate immediately with caramelized cherries, while filling is still soft.

CARAMELIZED CHERRIES

1) Mix together agave and lemon juice; fold in cherries. Blend well and let macerate for 1 hour.

2) Strain cherries and place on Teflex sheet; place into dehydrator at 110° for approximately 3 hours.

3) Cherries will be soft and well-glazed; cut cherries in half. Place cherries immediately on top of chocolate filling.

TO FINISH

1) Place decorated, cherry-topped torte into refrigerator for 4 hours.

2) When serving, use a chef's knife to cut the torte in half first, then cut each half into 6 evenly-cut slices. Run the knife under hot water and dry with a towel between slices so the knife will slice smoothly. Serve each slice with a sprig of mint.

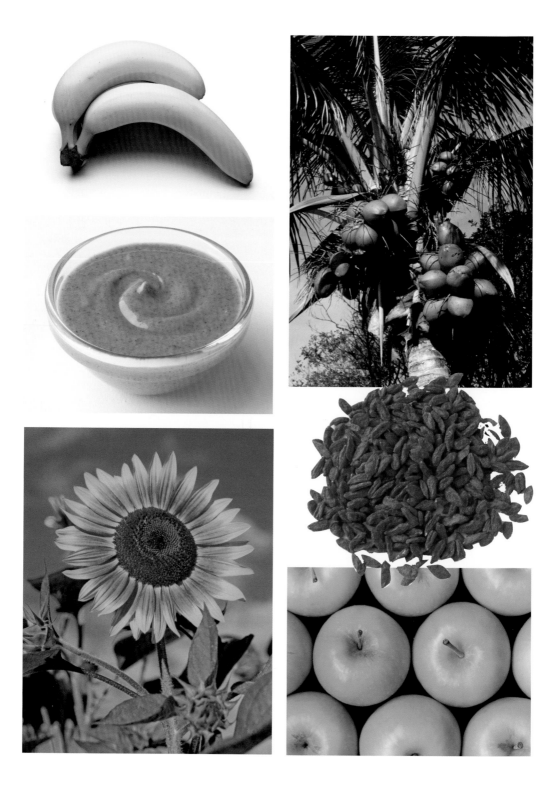

Goji Berry Vanilla Pudding

INGREDIENTS

3 tbsp water

1 tbsp coconut oil

1 tbsp almond butter

2 ripe bananas

1 tbsp goji berries (soaked for 10 minutes, drained, dehydrated for 6 hours)

2 tbsp lucuma powder

~~ vanilla powder

~~ banana slices

PREPARATION INSTRUCTIONS

1) Mix water and coconut with lucuma; add to blender.

2) Add all other ingredients except goji berries.

3) Blend until mixture becomes pudding texture.

4) Place goji berries into glasses.

5) Pour pudding over berries.

6) Garnish with vanilla powder and banana slices.

Green Apple Coconut Panna Cotta Granité

INGREDIENTS

½ cup fresh young coconut (or coconut flaked or shredded, soaked, then dried)

1 cup coconut milk

¼ cup prepared Irish moss

¼ cup white agave

¾ cup green apple puree

1 tsp fresh lemon juice

½ tsp coconut butter

~~ salt

PREPARATION INSTRUCTIONS

1) Soak Irish moss overnight and rinse 4 times until completely clean.

2) Blend all ingredients in blender on high speed until smooth.

3) Pour mixture into molds and freeze until set.

4) Remove from freezer; cut into chunks to fit into food processor. Pulse a few times to render to a granite consistency (somewhat like a frozen slush).

5) Serve immediately, garnished with a sauce, such as coulis of wild blueberry or guava tarragon glaze.

Guava Passion Fruit Custard with Star Anise and Strawberries

INGREDIENTS

1 cup fresh young Thai coconut, cut into small cubes (or coconut flakes, soaked and dried)

½ cup almond milk

2 ounces prepared Irish moss (per instructions on package)

¼ cup white agave

½ cup fresh or frozen passion fruit puree

½ cup fresh or frozen guava puree

1 star anise

PREPARATION INSTRUCTIONS

1) Place passion fruit puree in bowl – cover with plastic wrap – and put into bottom level of dehydrator.

2) Dehydrate at 115 degrees; reduce mixture to ⅓.

3) Prepare the guava puree in the same manner.

4) Mix the purees together; add the star anise to purees for 15 minutes to infuse flavor. Remove star anise.

5) Place all remaining ingredients into a blender, mix at high speed until mixture is completely smooth. Scrape sides as necessary.

6) Serve over fresh strawberries.

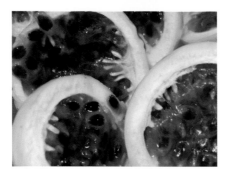

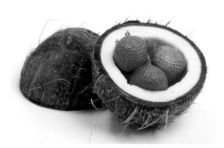

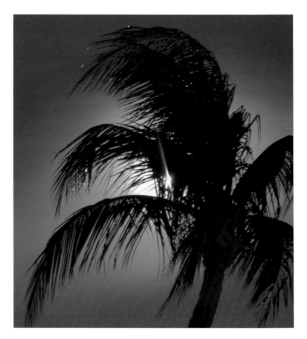

Key Lime Torte with Almond Date Crust

INGREDIENTS

9-INCH ALMOND DATE CRUST

3 cups almond flour

2 tsp agave

6 soft Medjool dates

2 tbsp coconut oil

~~ Himalayan sea salt

KEY LIME FILLING

6 ounces fresh key lime juice

1 ripe avocado, peeled, pitted, diced

½ ripe banana, peeled, diced

3 tbsp fresh mango, diced

¼ cup white agave

⅓ cup coconut butter

1 tsp vanilla extract

PREPARATION INSTRUCTIONS

ALMOND DATE CRUST

1) Place almond flour, dates, coconut oil and sea salt in food processor and blend until course and well mixed.

2) Press crust into 9-inch pie pan; dehydrate at 110° for 3½ hours. Remove and place in refrigerator.

KEY LIME FILLING

1) Put all filling ingredients, except coconut butter, in blender and blend on high speed until smooth and fluid.

2) Add coconut oil and blend until well finished.

3) Pour into crust and place in freezer for 3 hours.

TO FINISH

1) Cut into slices and serve with fresh berries or decorate with berry sauce.

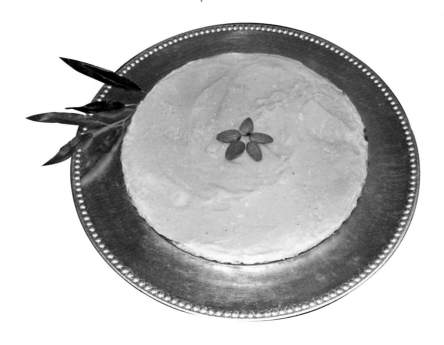

Kiwi Banana Chia Vanilla Pudding

INGREDIENTS

3 tbsp chia seeds

2 ounces coconut milk

2 ounces coconut water

1 cup ripe bananas
(peeled, diced)

1 tbsp vanilla powder
(or 1 tsp vanilla extract)

1 tsp agave

1 tsp fresh lemon juice

2 ounces Irish moss
(soaked overnight, washed till
clean and dried)

~~ dash Himalayan salt

PREPARATION INSTRUCTIONS

1) Soak chia seeds in the coconut water until they expand. (They will look like small, dark tapioca – if soaked overnight, they will be ready in the morning.)

2) Put all ingredients into blender and blend on high speed until mixture is smooth.

3) Place mixture into the refrigerator until it is set and has the consistency of pudding.

4) Serve in a martini glass, garnished with kiwi.

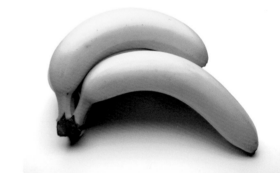

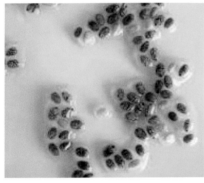

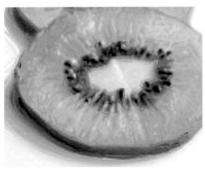

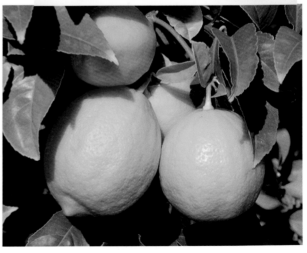

Macadamia-Mango Delight with Coulis of Wild Blueberry

INGREDIENTS

MACADAMIA-MANGO DELIGHT

1 cup macadamia nuts, soaked for 4 hours and dehydrated for 6 hours

1 tbsp coconut oil, warmed to liquefy

¼ cup Irish moss, soaked for 15 minutes and drained

¼ cup agave

1 cup sliced, peeled ripe mangoes

WILD BLUEBERRY COULIS

1 cup wild blueberries

1 tsp agave

1 tsp fresh lemon juice

2 tbsp cold water

4 ounces coconut milk (see recipe included in package)

~~ sea salt

PREPARATION INSTRUCTIONS

MACADAMIA-MANGO DELIGHT

1) Place macadamia nuts and coconut oil in a food processor and process until smooth.

2) Place the nut/oil mixture into a blender and add in the remaining ingredients.

3) Blend on high speed until very smooth.

4) Pour into glasses.

WILD BLUEBERRY COULIS

1) Place all ingredients into a blender and mix on high speed until smooth.

2) Put coulis mixture into a pan and place on the bottom of the dehydrator.

3) Reduce until mixture coats a spoon.

4) Garnish the macadamia-mango delight with the coulis.

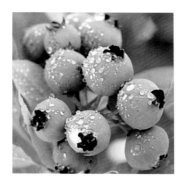 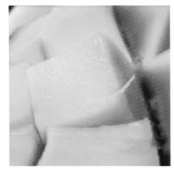 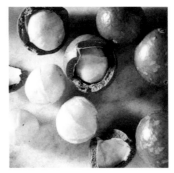

Mango Gelato

INGREDIENTS

½ cup fresh young coconut (or coconut flaked or shredded, soaked, then dried)

1 cup coconut milk

¼ cup prepared Irish moss

¼ cup white agave

¾ cup mango, peeled, diced

1 tsp fresh lemon juice

½ tsp coconut butter

~~ salt

PREPARATION INSTRUCTIONS

1) Soak Irish moss overnight and rinse 4 times until completely clean.

2) Blend all ingredients in blender on high speed until smooth.

3) Pour mixture into molds and freeze until set.

4) Remove from freezer until gelato softens to the correct frosty, creamy consistency — when it is easy to scoop.

5) Garnish with dark chocolate fudge sauce.

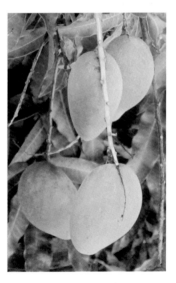
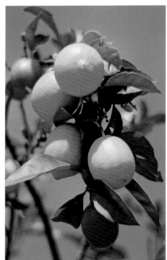
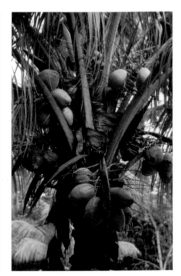

Mixed Berry and Vanilla Peach Dreams with Macadamia Nut Clouds

INGREDIENTS

MIXED BERRY AND VANILLA PEACH DREAMS

2 fresh peaches

~ mixed berries, amount to liking

1 tbsp maple syrup

½ tsp cinnamon powder

~ fresh lime juice to taste

1 tsp vanilla powder or ½ tsp vanilla extract

MACADAMIA NUT CLOUDS

1 cup macadamia nuts

~ water to cover nuts

1 tbsp agave

PREPARATION INSTRUCTIONS

1) Cut peaches in half; remove pit, then cut each peach into 8 slices for a total of 16 slices.

2) Place peach slices in a marinade of the maple syrup, vanilla, lime juice and cinnamon; marinate for 1 hour. Drain and place peaches on a Teflex sheet and dehydrate at 115° until tender. Cool, then blend with mixed berries; set aside.

3) Place macadamia nuts into high speed blender; add enough water to cover nuts. Blend until texture is that of cream cheese.

4) Place cheese cloth over a sieve, place sieve over a large bowl; put nut mixture into cheese cloth. Close cloth around nut mixture, place a plate and a weight on top of sieve. Put in warm place for 14 hours to allow mixture to drain off excess water.

5) Put nut mixture into a bowl and mix in agave; refrigerate until mixture sets up to a cream cheese consistency.

6) Place peach and berry mixture into glasses; top with macadamia nut clouds.

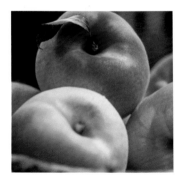
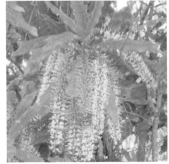
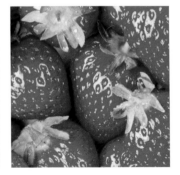

Pina Colada Frosty Treats

INGREDIENTS

1½ cups pineapple, finely diced (one cup will be used to make pineapple concentrate; the other ½ cup will be held for inclusion at end of preparation.)

2 tbsp shredded coconut

1½ cup coconut milk

4 tbsp agave

1 tsp vanilla extract

2 tbsp lime juice

PREPARATION INSTRUCTIONS

PINEAPPLE CONCENTRATE

1) Place 1 cup finely diced pineapple on Teflex sheet and dehydrate at 110° for 2 hours. Remove; put dehydrated pineapple into blender and blend on high speed for 15 seconds.

2) Put crushed pineapple in pan or bowl and place on bottom of dehydrator. Dehydrate at 115° until pineapple is reduced to a syrup. One cup of pineapple should reduce down to ½ cup of pineapple concentrate.

FROSTY TREATS

1) Place coconut milk, agave, vanilla extract, lime juice and pineapple concentrate into a blender and blend well.

2) Pour into ice cream maker and follow manufacturer's directions.

3) Just before the end of the ice cream making cycle, add the remaining ½ cup fresh, finely diced pineapple and the shredded coconut.

4) When well blended and frozen to the correct consistency, remove and store in freezer.

NOTE:

You may enjoy this ice cream from a bowl, rolled into balls and coated with shredded coconut like a bon-bon, or put into a popsicle mold to create a frosty treat on a stick.

Pumpkin Mousse

INGREDIENTS

1¾ cup pumpkin, pared, diced

½ ripe banana

½ cup prepared Irish moss gel

½ cup coconut milk

¼ cup coconut water

½ tbsp coconut butter

½ cup almond milk

¼ tsp nutmeg

2 tbsp coconut palm sugar

1½ tsp cinnamon powder

~~ sea salt

PREPARATION INSTRUCTIONS

1) Prepare Irish moss to package instructions to yield ½ cup gel, usually soaked overnight.

2) Flavor diced pumpkin with small amount of coconut butter, palm sugar, nutmeg and cinnamon (measured ingredients listed above are for main recipe).

3) Place flavored pumpkin pieces on Teflex sheet and dehydrate for 2 hours at 105°.

4) Place all ingredients, including pumpkin, into blender and blend until smooth. Pour into glass bowl and cover; place in refrigerator to set.

5) To serve, put mousse into martini glasses and top with candied pecans.

NOTE:

To make a parfait, layer pumpkin mouse with vanilla ice cream, crushed candied pecans and top with 1 candied pecan half.

Spicy Cherries

INGREDIENTS

1 cup dried raw cherries

¼ tsp five spice powder

2 tbsp maple syrup

¼ tsp curry powder

~~ touch cayenne powder

PREPARATION INSTRUCTIONS

1) Soak cherries until soft, approximately 2 hours; drain and dry between paper towels.

2) Mix together maple syrup, five spice powder and cayenne.

3) When well blended, add cherries and coat completely.

4) Let cherries stand in marinade for 15 minutes.

5) Place cherries onto Teflex sheet and dehydrate for 6 hours.

Vanilla Mint Ice Cream

INGREDIENTS

VANILLA MINT ICE CREAM

1 cup coconut water

1½ cups almond milk

¼ cup chopped coconut meat or coconut flakes, soaked for 1 hour and drained

2 tbsp coconut oil

½ tbsp vanilla extract

3 tbsp fresh mint leaves

¼ tsp mint extract

¼ cup date paste

DATE PASTE

1 cup pitted Barhi dates*

½ cup water

PREPARATION INSTRUCTIONS

VANILLA MINT ICE CREAM

1) In blender, combine and blend date paste, coconut water, almond milk, coconut meat, coconut oil, and vanilla extract. Process at high speed until smooth.

2) Transfer to a bowl and add the minced mint leaves.

3) Freeze in an ice cream maker, according to the manufacturer's directions. Add the mint extract to the ice cream at the last 3 turns.

Serve with dehydrated slices of fresh fruit.

DATE PASTE

1) Soak the dates for 1 hour in cold water.

2) Remove water, pressing out by hand.

3) Combine the dates and water in a food processor; process until completely smooth.

Use immediately or store in a covered glass container, in the refrigerator, for up to 12 days.

*Barhi dates are the sweetest and softest of all dates; when frozen they taste like caramel candy.

Wake Me Shake Me Chocolate Coffee Mousse

INGREDIENTS

1 avocado, pitted and peeled

3 tbsp raw cocoa powder

2 tbsp dehydrated coffee, ground to the same consistency as the cocoa powder

¼ cup water

¼ cup agave

1 tsp vanilla extract

1 tsp cinnamon

PREPARATION INSTRUCTIONS

1) Put all ingredients in blender and puree on high speed until mixture is completely smooth, stopping to scrape the sides as necessary.

2) Serve in a martini glass.

3) Garnish with almond brittle crunch.

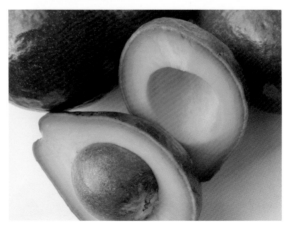

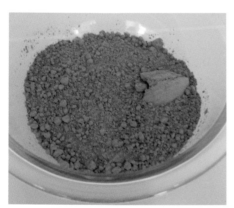

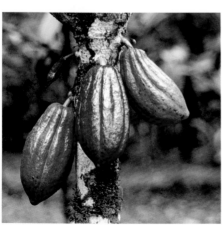

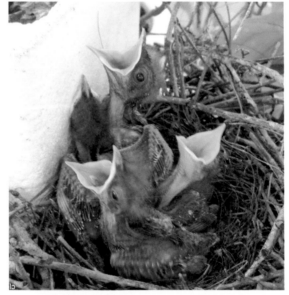

Dips, etc.

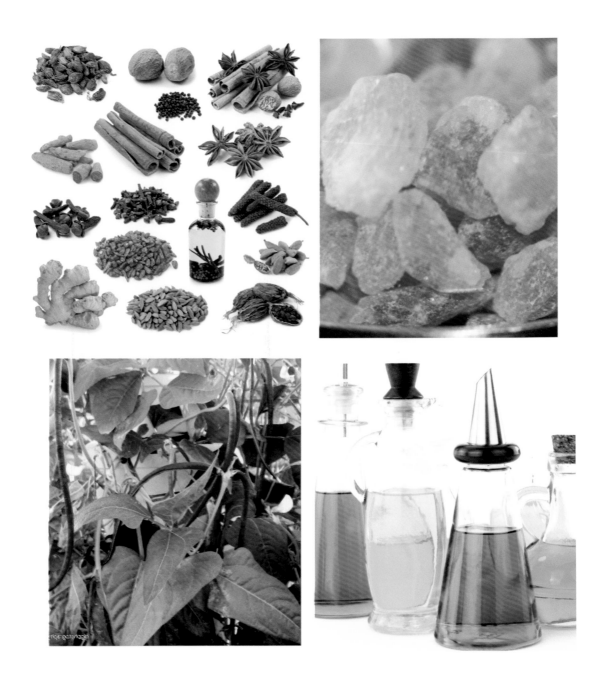

Barhi Date Paste

INGREDIENTS

1 cup pitted Barhi dates*

½ cup water

PREPARATION INSTRUCTIONS

1) Soak the dates for 1 hour in cold water.

2) Remove water, pressing out by hand.

3) Combine the dates and water in a food processor; process until completely smooth.

Use immediately or store in a covered glass container, in the refrigerator, for up to 12 days.

*Barhi dates are the sweetest and softest of all dates; when frozen they taste like caramel candy.

Cilantro Curry Hummus

INGREDIENTS

1 cup sesame seeds (soaked 1 hour and dried)

1 cup pine nuts (soaked 1 hour and dried)

2 tbsp extra virgin olive oil

2 tbsp cold water

1 tbsp nama shoyu

½ tbsp agave

2 tbsp fresh lemon juice

2 tbsp chopped cilantro

1½ tbsp garlic powder

1 tbsp curry powder

1 tsp nutritional yeast

1 tsp Herbamare

~~ cayenne to taste

PREPARATION INSTRUCTIONS

1) Crush sesame seeds and pine nuts in blender; continue blending until smooth.

2) Add all other ingredients except olive oil and cilantro. Slowly add oil when mixture is well blended.

3) Put mixture in bowl and add chopped cilantro; flavor with salt and cayenne.

Coulis of Wild Blueberry

INGREDIENTS

1 cup wild blueberries

1 tsp agave

1 tsp fresh lemon juice

2 tbsp cold water

PREPARATION INSTRUCTIONS

1) Place all ingredients into a blender and mix on high speed until smooth.

2) Put coulis mixture into a pan and place on the bottom of the dehydrator.

3) Reduce until mixture coats a spoon.

Hummus, Basic Recipe

INGREDIENTS

1 cup sesame seeds
(soaked 1 hour and dried)

1 cup pine nuts
(soaked 1 hour and dried)

2 tbsp extra virgin olive oil

2 tbsp cold water

1 tbsp nama shoyu

2 tbsp fresh lemon juice

1½ tbsp garlic powder

1 tsp nutritional yeast

1 tsp Herbamare

½ tbsp agave

~~ cayenne to taste

PREPARATION INSTRUCTIONS

1) Crush sesame seeds and pine nuts in blender; continue blending until smooth.

2) Add all other ingredients except olive oil. Slowly add oil when mixture is well blended.

3) Put mixture in bowl and flavor with salt and cayenne.

Mint Citrus Almond Chutney

INGREDIENTS

6 ounces fresh mint, chopped

12 ounces almonds, soaked for 12 hours.

zest of 1 orange

zest of 1 lime

zest of 1 lemon

1 tsp Himalayan salt

1 tbsp fresh grated ginger

4 ounces orange juice

4 ounces raw agave

8 ounces extra virgin olive oil

PREPARATION INSTRUCTIONS

1) Put almonds in blender and pulse/chop.

2) Put all other ingredients into blender and pulse 4 times.

3) Add almonds to mixture and pulse a couple of times to blend well.

NOTE:

Great as a garnish for soups, salads and entrees.

Moo-Less Macadamia Cheese (Basic Recipe)

INGREDIENTS

1 cup macadamia nuts

~ water to cover nuts

1 tsp garlic powder

1 tsp onion powder

~ salt and pepper to taste

PREPARATION INSTRUCTIONS

1) Place macadamia nuts into high speed blender; add enough water to cover nuts. Blend until texture is that of cream cheese.

2) Place cheese cloth over a sieve, place sieve over a large bowl; put nut mixture into cheese cloth. Close cloth around nut mixture; place a plate and a weight on top of sieve. Put in warm place for 14 hours to allow mixture to drain off excess water.

3) Put nut mixture into a bowl and mix in onion powder, garlic powder and salt and pepper to taste; refrigerate until mixture sets up to a cream cheese consistency.

NOTE:

The above recipe is for basic cheese. Depending on your use, you can blend in any variety of fresh herbs, spices, minced vegetable or fruits.

Rosemary Thyme Herb Hummus

INGREDIENTS

1 cup sesame seeds
(soaked for 1 hour and dried)

1 cup pine nuts
(soaked for 1 hour and dried)

2 tbsp Salba oil

2 tbsp cold water

1 tbsp nama shoyu

½ tbsp agave

2 tbsp fresh lemon juice

1 tbsp thyme, finely chopped

1½ tbsp garlic powder

1 tbsp rosemary,
finely chopped

1 tsp nutritional yeast

1 tsp Herbamare

~ salt and cayenne to taste

PREPARATION INSTRUCTIONS

1) Crush sesame seeds and pine nuts in blender; continue blending until smooth.

2) Add all other ingredients except oil, thyme and rosemary. Slowly add oils until mixture is well blended.

3) Put mixture in bowl and add chopped thyme and rosemary. Flavor with salt and cayenne.

4) Set aside for future use.

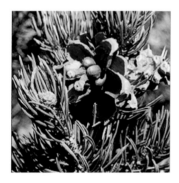
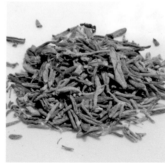
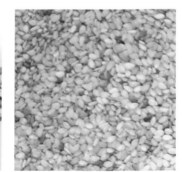

Sal's Almond Butter

INGREDIENTS

3 cups raw almonds
(do not soak)

¾ cup red palm oil

1 tbsp agave

1 tsp cinnamon powder

1 tsp sea salt

~~ touch cayenne

PREPARATION INSTRUCTIONS

1) Place almonds in blender and blend on low speed until they become a flour-like texture.

2) Turn blender up to high speed and add salt, cayenne, agave and cinnamon.

3) Very slowly add palm oil into mixture through top of blender, until it reaches the consistency of butter.

4) Store in glass jar in refrigerator.

NOTE:

The process of adding the oil slowly into the almond mixture will take some time. Keep constant vigil on attaining the consistency you like.

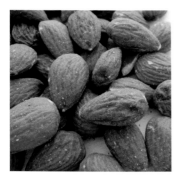
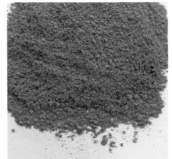
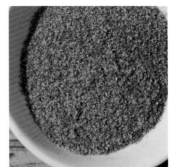

Dressings

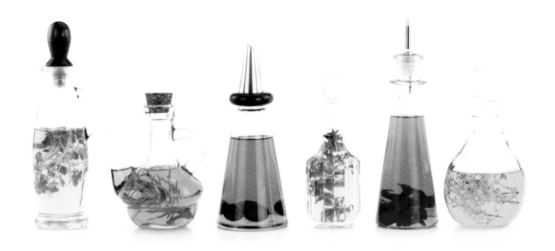

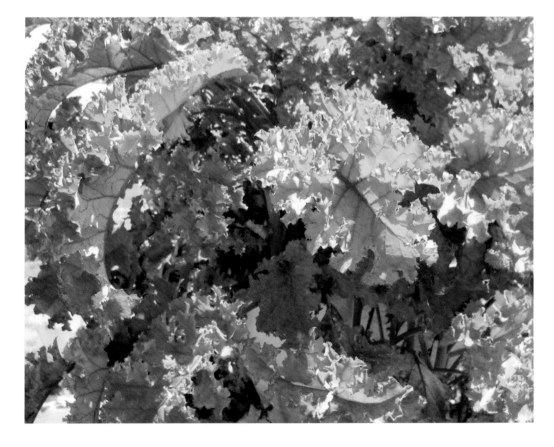

Asian Dressing

INGREDIENTS

6 tbsp raw tahini
(sesame seeds, sea salt)

1 ¼ cup cold water

¾ cup green onions, diced

2 tbsp flaxseed oil

2 tbsp sesame seed oil

1 tbsp grape seed oil

1 tbsp maple syrup

3 tbsp ginger, peeled
and grated

½ tsp cayenne

1 tbsp nama shoyu

½ tsp cumin

~~ coconut flakes

PREPARATION INSTRUCTIONS

1) Add all ingredients to blender, blending on high speed until smooth. If necessary, dilute by adding water.

2) Serve over mixed greens, with carrots, celery, sprouts, daikon, radishes, parsley.

3) Just before serving, add coconut flakes.

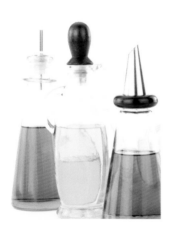
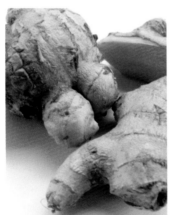
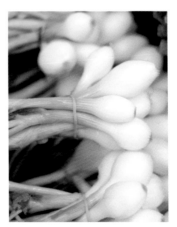

Avocado Dressing

INGREDIENTS

1 ripe avocado

6 tbsp cold water

1 tsp white miso

1 tsp onion powder

1 tsp garlic powder

1 tsp Himalayan sea salt

1 tbsp fresh lemon juice

½ cup olive oil

PREPARATION INSTRUCTIONS

1) Add all ingredients to blender except olive oil, blending on high speed until smooth.

2) While still on high speed, slowly add olive oil to mixture. Blend until dressing is a creamy consistency.

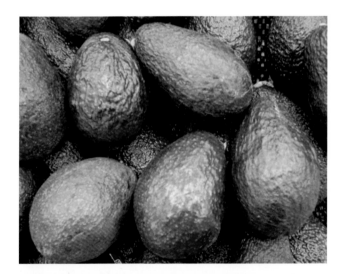

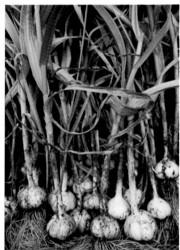

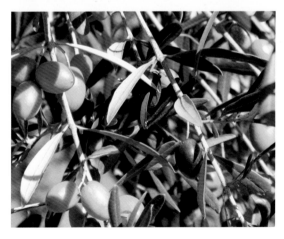

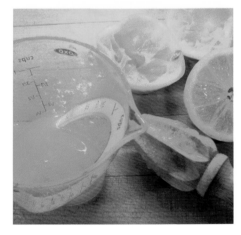

Chestnut Vinaigrette

INGREDIENTS

½ cup soft chestnuts, clean-prepped*

¼ cup dates, soaked 1 hour, drained, cut in quarters

¼ cup dark grapes, cut in half

¾ cup red palm oil

¼ cup apple cider vinegar

¼ cup warm water

1 tsp pomegranate molasses

¼ tsp garlic powder

¼ tsp onion powder

~~ salt to taste

PREPARATION INSTRUCTIONS

1) Place all ingredients into food processor.
2) Blend until very fine.
3) Strain and store in glass jar in refrigerator.

NOTE:

*To clean-prep chestnuts, wash, dry, remove any dark skins.

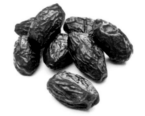

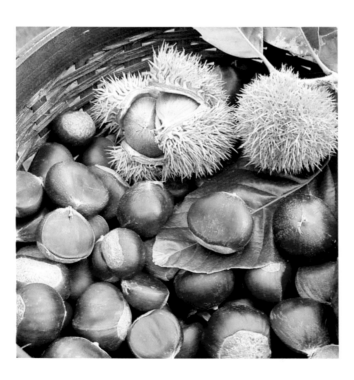

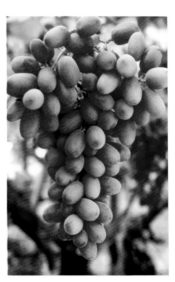

Herb Vinaigrette Dressing

INGREDIENTS

2 tbsp apple cider vinegar

6 tbsp extra virgin olive oil

1 tbsp maple syrup

1 tbsp mustard

½ tsp fresh Italian parsley, chopped

½ tsp fresh thyme, chopped

½ tsp fresh basil, chopped

½ tsp fresh garlic, chopped very fine

1 tbsp cold water, if needed

~~ sea salt and pepper to taste

PREPARATION INSTRUCTIONS

1) Add all ingredients to blender, blending on high speed. Dilute, if necessary, with water.

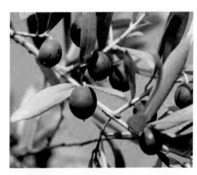

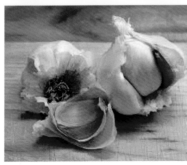

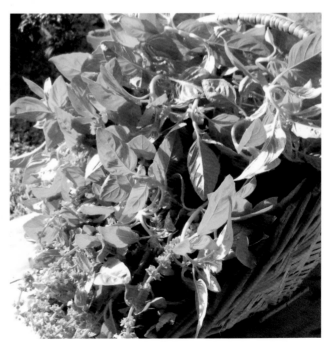

Mango Vinaigrette

INGREDIENTS

½ cup fresh diced mango

2 tbsp maple syrup

3 tbsp apple cider vinegar

1 cup grape seed oil

1 tbsp fresh lemon juice

1 tsp cold water

~~ salt, to taste

~~ cayenne, to taste

¼ cup fresh mango, minced, at end

1 tbsp fresh mint, minced, at end

PREPARATION INSTRUCTIONS

1) In blender add all ingredients, except water. Blend well.

2) Add water, blend briefly.

3) To finish, gently mix in minced mango and mint.

Miso Lemon Dressing

INGREDIENTS

1 tbsp white miso

1 tsp fresh ginger, peeled, diced

1 tbsp nama shoyu

1 whole lemon, cut in pieces

1 tbsp maple syrup

2 tbsp apple cider vinegar

touch chili powder

½ cup extra virgin olive oil

¼ cup cold water

PREPARATION INSTRUCTIONS

1) Add all ingredients to blender, blending on high speed until smooth. (Keep cold water aside.) If necessary, dilute by adding water.

Salads

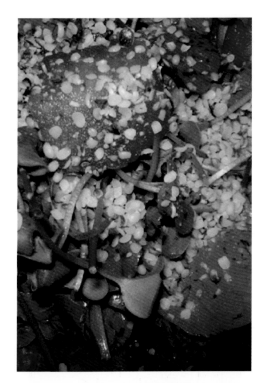

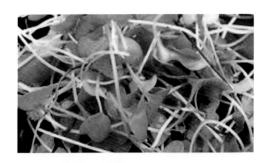

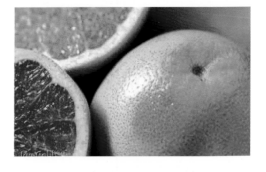

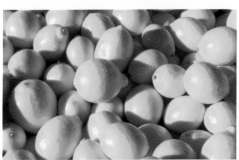

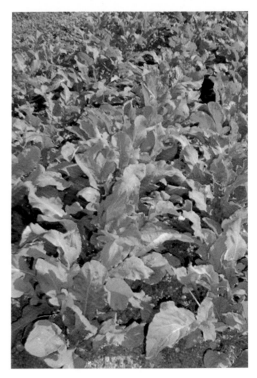

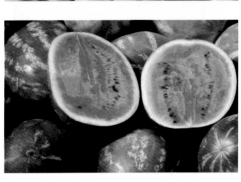

Arugula, Micro Greens Salad with Grapefruit Segments and Watermelon Squares in Lemon, Grape Seed Oil Vinaigrette

INGREDIENTS

SALAD INGREDIENTS PER PERSON

3 ounces arugula and micro greens mixture

5 medium diced fresh watermelon squares

5 fresh grapefruit segments, dehydrated on Teflex sheet for 30 minutes

1 tsp hemp hearts

VINAIGRETTE

¼ cup fresh squeezed and strained lemon juice

1 lemon, finely zested

1 tbs raw agave

1 tsp Himalayan sea salt

½ cup grape seed oil

PREPARATION INSTRUCTIONS

1) Put all ingredients, except oil, in blender on high speed. Add oil very slowly to finish vinaigrette.

2) Place arugula and micro greens mixture in bowl and toss with vinaigrette; remove greens to individual plates.

3) Place grapefruit segments and diced watermelon squares into the bowl that held the greens mixture. Coat fruit with vinaigrette.

4) Top greens with vinaigrette-coated fruit.

5) Garnish salad with hemp hearts.

Beet-Carrot Salad

INGREDIENTS

2 medium-sized beets, cleaned, dark ends/stems removed

5 carrots, cleaned, dark ends and stems removed

2 large cloves of garlic, peeled

½ cup apple cider vinegar

1 tsp ground cinnamon

1 tbsp raw white agave

1 tsp Himalayan sea salt

½ cup grape seed oil

1 tbsp ginger, peeled and diced

~~ pinch cayenne

PREPARATION INSTRUCTIONS

1) Place vegetables in food processor and chop all vegetables to medium-sized chunks.

2) Add half of all ingredients, except the grape seed oil in food processor. Pulse until mixture is a bit finer consistency, but still coarse.

3) Add ¼ cup of grape seed oil to this batch and set aside.

4) Do the same with the remaining half of ingredients. Place in food processor and pulse until mixture is a bit finer consistency, but still coarse. Add the remaining ¼ cup of grape seed oil to this mixture.

5) Mix both batches together and store in a glass container until use.

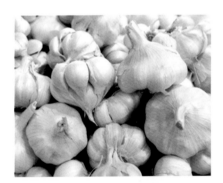
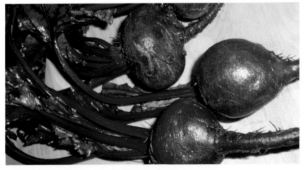
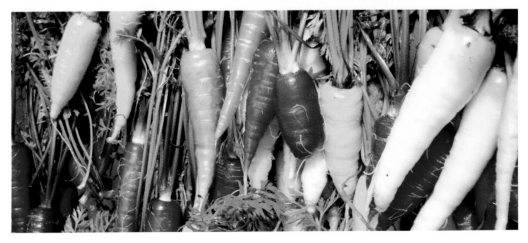

Chunky Cherry Grapefruit Relish

INGREDIENTS

1 cup cherries, fresh or frozen

1 red grapefruit

~~ agave, to taste

2 tsp lemon zest

PREPARATION INSTRUCTIONS

1) Pit cherries and cut each into 4 pieces.

2) Remove segments from grapefruit; cut each segment into 4 pieces.

3) Toss cherries and grapefruit together to mix.

4) Serve topped with a sprinkling of lemon zest.

NOTE:

Depending on sweetness or tartness of grapefruit, you may choose to add a drop or two of agave.

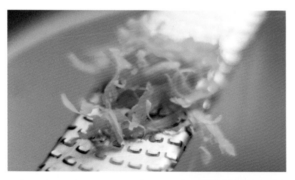

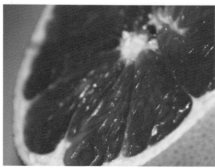
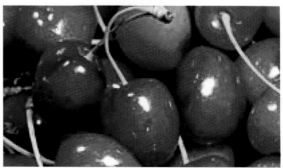

Curry Spring Salad with Spicy Pecans

INGREDIENTS

SALAD

shredded green cabbage

julienne red pepper

julienne nasturtium greens

diced papaya

diced pineapple

julienne carrots

julienne red onion

diced avocado

CURRY SAUCE

1 tbsp curry powder

1 tsp turmeric

1 tsp coriander

1 tsp cumin

1 cup coconut milk

1 tbsp fresh ginger juice

1 tbsp agave

~ salt to taste

~ dash cayenne

PREPARATION INSTRUCTIONS

CURRY SAUCE

1) Put all ingredients into blender and blend until smooth.

2) Place in bowl; cover with plastic wrap.

3) Place on bottom of dehydrator at 115 degrees till reduced by ⅓.

TO SERVE

1) Soak handful of raisins in a coconut water/garam masala mixture; drain, dehydrate 4 hours at 110°.

2) Mix salad with curry sauce.

3) Garnish with mint almond chutney and flavored raisins.

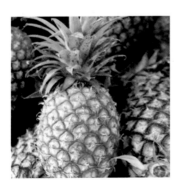
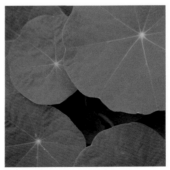
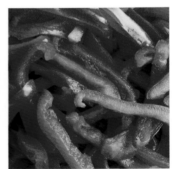

Fennel, Arugula, Apple and Pomegranate Salad

INGREDIENTS

DRESSING

¼ cup extra virgin olive oil

2 tbsp fresh lemon juice

3 tbsp apple cider vinegar

3 ounces red onion, small diced

seeds of ½ fresh pomegranate

1 tbsp agave

enough fresh arugula per salad/per person

VEGETABLE/FRUIT/NUT MIXTURE

1 small fennel, medium diced

handful of pecans, rough chopped

seeds of ½ fresh pomegranate

salt and pepper to taste

2 Fuji or Pink Lady apples, medium diced

PREPARATION INSTRUCTIONS

1) Mix all dressing ingredients in blender.

2) In large bowl, mix together all other ingredients except arugula.

3) Mix arugula with dressing and place on individual salad plates. Top with vegetable/fruit/nut mixture.

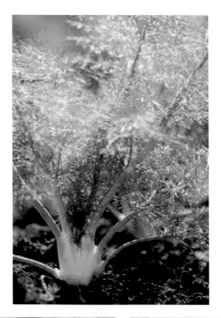

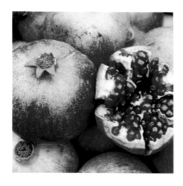

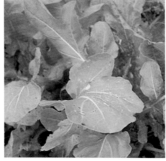

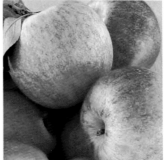

Golden Beet Tartare

INGREDIENTS

4 ounces golden beets

1 tbsp cucumber

1 tbsp mango

1 tbsp avocado

1 tbsp miso vinaigrette

~~ sea salt, to taste

~~ cilantro

PREPARATION INSTRUCTIONS

1) Peel beets and cut into ¼ inch slices. Dice small.

2) Peel the cucumber, mango, and avocado; dice all the same size as beets.

3) Toss all ingredients together, except cilantro.

4) Season with salt and miso vinaigrette. Toss to mix well.

5) Garnish with cilantro.

SERVING SUGGESTION:

Pair golden beet tartare together with red beet tartare, side by side, as a salad or as an accompaniment to an entrée.

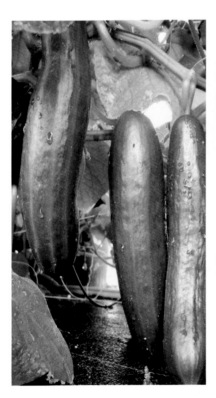

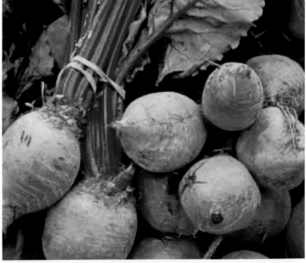

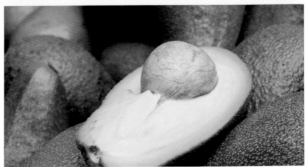

Granny Smith's Apple Stuffing

INGREDIENTS

2 Granny Smith apples with skin on

¼ cup minced celery

2 tbsp fresh lime juice

1 tbsp lime zest

2 tbsp white agave

1 tsp cinnamon powder

~~ Bell's poultry seasoning

PREPARATION INSTRUCTIONS

1) Core apples and small dice.

2) Peel celery to remove strings; slice through celery very thinly, then mince very small.

3) Put all ingredients, except celery, in bowl and mix well.

4) Place on Teflex sheet and dehydrate at 105° for 1½ hours.

5) Remove from dehydrator and put all ingredients from sheet into food processor; using "S" blade, pulse a few times until apple is coarsely chopped.

6) Finish by putting apple mixture into bowl and add in minced celery; stir well.

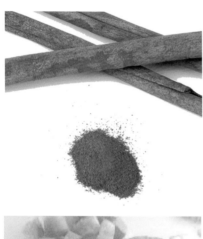

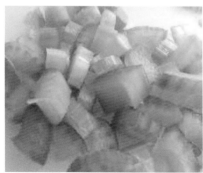

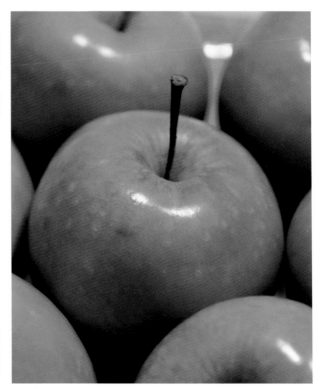

Hemp Hearts Spring Salad

INGREDIENTS

½ lb fresh spinach leaves

6 fresh nasturtium leaves

1 avocado, diced

1 grapefruit, cut into segments, retain juice

1 apple with skin, diced

4 ounces grape seed oil

3 tbsp hemp hearts per person

~~ touch of sea salt

cayenne to taste

PREPARATION INSTRUCTIONS

1) Blend all juice from grapefruit with grape seed oil and salt; set aside.

2) Mix spinach with nasturtium leaves; add avocado, grapefruit segments and apple.

3) Toss with grapefruit juice/oil dressing.

4) Garnish with hemp hearts.

5) Add touch of cayenne if desired.

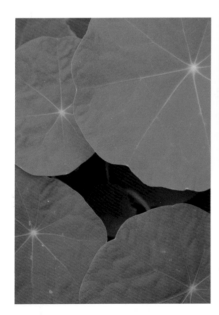

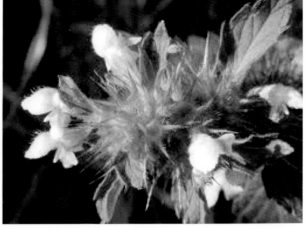

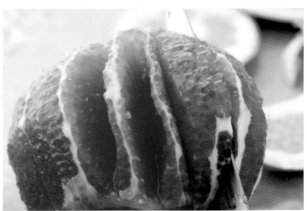

Japanese Sea Vegetable Salad with Cherries

INGREDIENTS

1 cup dried cherries, soaked in water for 1 hour, drained and dried

1 ounce dried wakame

1 ounce dried hijiki

1 ounce dried arame

½ sheet dried nori sea vegetable

2 tbsp white sesame seeds

2 tbsp black sesame seeds

1 large cucumber, peeled, seeded and julienned

1 large beet, peeled and julienned

1 medium daikon radish, peeled and julienned

1 green onion, bulb and 1 inch of the green, sliced very thin

~~ cayenne to taste

PREPARATION INSTRUCTIONS

1) In separate bowls, soak the sea vegetables in water until soft. Wait 10 minutes to drain water. The hijiki and wakame may take up to 20 minutes.

2) Drain the sea vegetables, using your hands, squeeze out as much water as possible. Roughly chop the wakame into smaller pieces.

3) Place the sea vegetables in a large bowl; add the cucumber, beets, radish and dried cherries.

4) Pour Miso Lemon Dressing onto vegetables and toss gently to combine.

5) Sprinkle with green onion, black and white sesame seeds; add a small dash of cayenne, if desired.

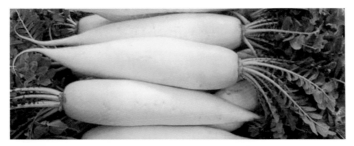

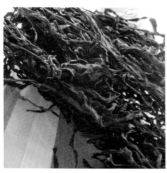
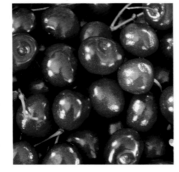
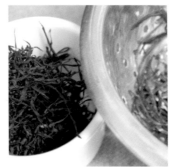

Jicama Confetti Salad

INGREDIENTS

5 ounces jicama

2 ounces red bell pepper

2 ounces mango meat,
ripe but firm

2 ounces red cabbage

2 ounces carrots

~~ sea salt to taste

~~ vinaigrette of choice

PREPARATION INSTRUCTIONS

1) Peel and julienne jicama, mango and carrots. Put in bowl.

2) Core and seed red bell pepper; cut into julienne strips. Add to bowl.

3) Remove outer leaves of cabbage and cut into julienne strips. Add to bowl.

4) Flavor with sea salt.

5) Toss everything together with vinaigrette.

6) To serve, arrange julienne strips on middle of plates and top with parsley.

NOTE:

Either Asian or chestnut vinaigrettes are great with this salad. For an extra punch of color, drizzle red palm oil around the salad.

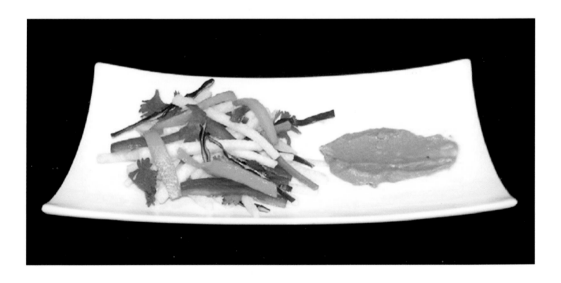

Petite Salad of Arugula with Sweet & Sour Red Onions and Herb Vinaigrette

INGREDIENTS

HERB VINAIGRETTE

2 tbsp apple cider vinegar

6 tbsp extra virgin olive oil

1 tbsp maple syrup

1 tbsp mustard

½ tsp fresh, chopped Italian parsley

½ tsp fresh, chopped thyme

½ tsp fresh, chopped basil

½ tsp fresh garlic, chopped fine

1 tbsp cold water, if needed

~ salt and pepper to taste

SWEET & SOUR RED ONIONS

1 red onion, peeled, cut into small slices

2 tbsp apple cider vinegar

1 tbsp maple syrup

½ tsp sea salt

PETITE SALAD

small handful of fresh arugula per person

PREPARATION INSTRUCTIONS

HERB VINAIGRETTE

1) Put all ingredients in blender, blending on high speed. Dilute, if necessary, with water.

SWEET & SOUR RED ONIONS

1) Peel red onion; cut into small slices. Place into bowl and add apple cider vinegar, sea salt, and maple syrup. Marinate for 3 hours. Drain and dehydrate on Teflex sheet at 115° until tender.

TO FINISH SALAD

1) Wash and thoroughly dry fresh arugula; remove any long stems. Toss arugula into herb vinaigrette. Put small handful of greens on middle of small plate.

2) Place mound of sweet & sour red onions on top of arugula.

Red Beet Carpaccio with Ginger

INGREDIENTS

2 small beets

1 tbsp shallots

3 tbsp extra virgin olive oil

3 tbsp apple cider vinegar

1 tsp ginger

1 tsp garlic

fresh chives

~~ sea salt and freshly ground pepper

PREPARATION INSTRUCTIONS

1) Peel the beets and slice very thinly. Use a Japanese mandoline for best results.

2) Peel garlic and mince. Peel shallots and mince.

3) Combine beets, shallots, ginger, garlic, olive oil and apple cider vinegar in a bowl. Toss to mix and season with salt and pepper.

TO SERVE:

Arrange sliced beets on a plate, overlapping the slices. Spoon remaining liquid over the beets and garnish with fresh chives.

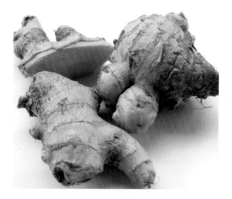
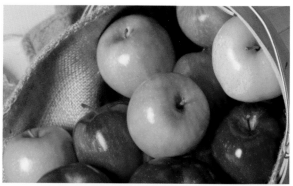
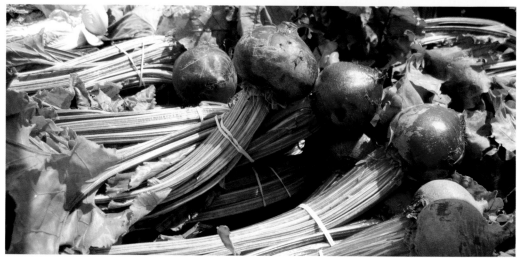

Sea and Land Asian Salad

INGREDIENTS

½ ounce dried wakame

½ ounce dried hijiki

½ ounce dried arame

½ ounce nori

8 ounces fresh young Thai coconut meat **

1 medium daikon, peeled and julienned

½ cup fresh radishes, sliced and julienned

4 small handfuls of assorted fresh, spicy Asian greens

1 small cucumber, peeled, seeded and julienned

PREPARATION INSTRUCTIONS

1) Soak arame and nori in cold water for about 5 to 10 minutes until soft.

2) Soak wakame and hijiki for up to 20 minutes until soft.

3) Drain sea vegetables and squeeze out as much of the water as possible.

4) Roughly chop wakame and nori into smaller pieces.

5) Place all sea vegetables in a large bowl. Add the remainder of the vegetables and toss gently.

6) Mix well with Miso Lemon Dressing.

7) Garnish with spicy cherries and sprinkle with white sesame seeds.

** If fresh young Thai coconut meat is not available, use dried, shredded coconut and soak in water for 1 hour prior to using.

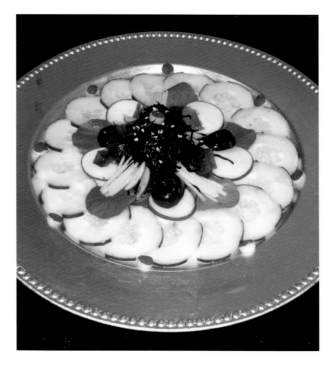

Tartare of Red Beets

INGREDIENTS

4 ounces red beets
1 tbsp red onion
1 tsp ginger, grated
1 tbsp red palm oil
1 tsp apple cider vinegar
~~ sea salt, to taste

PREPARATION INSTRUCTIONS

1) Peel beets and cut into ¼ inch slices. Dice small.

2) Dice red onion to same size as beets.

3) Toss all ingredients together, including grated ginger.

4) Season with salt, vinegar and red palm oil. Toss to mix well.

SERVING SUGGESTION:

Pair red beet tartare together with golden beet tartare, side by side, as a salad or as an accompaniment to an entrée.

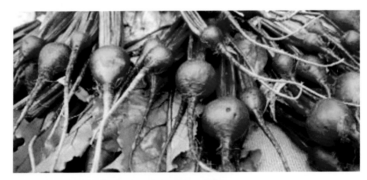

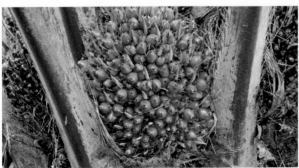

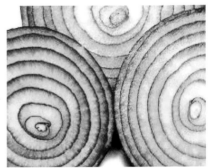

Tropical Pineapple Salsa

INGREDIENTS

½ cup fresh pineapple

½ cup fresh mango

¼ cup fresh coconut

1 tsp red onion

1 tbsp fresh cilantro

2 tbsp lime juice

~~ salt and pepper to taste

PREPARATION INSTRUCTIONS

1) Peel pineapple and mango, cut into small dice.

2) Remove meat from coconut, cut into small dice.

3) Wash, dry, and remove stems from cilantro. Chop very fine.

4) Peel onion and mince.

5) Mix together in bowl.

6) Add lime juice and salt and pepper to taste. Mix well.

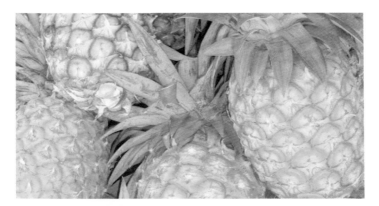

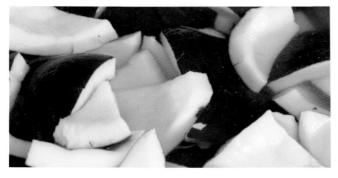

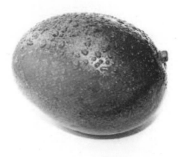

Sauces

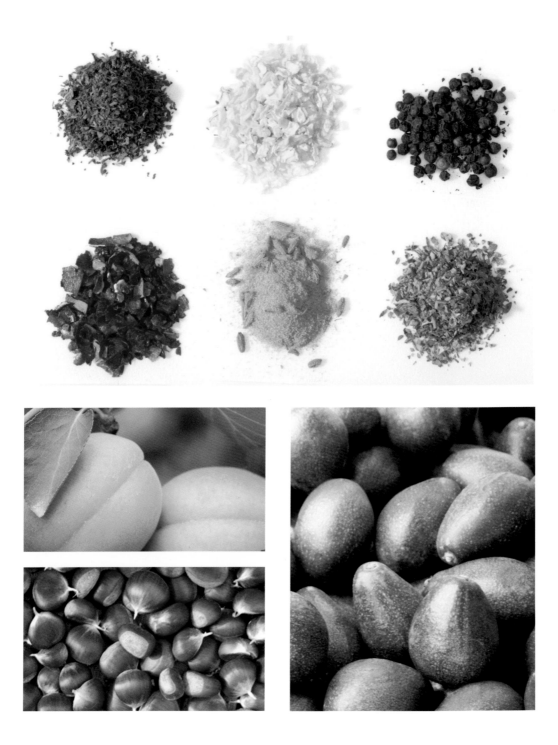

Apricot Barbecue Sauce

INGREDIENTS

6 dried apricots

1 chipotle pepper, seeds removed, large diced

1 cup red pepper, cored, seeds removed, large diced

1 large shallot, peeled, small diced

1 tbsp fresh garlic, peeled, small diced

⅓ cup maple syrup

⅓ cup apple cider vinegar

1 tsp ground chili powder

1 tsp ground cumin

1 tsp ground paprika powder

1 tsp Himalayan sea salt

1 tbsp maca

PREPARATION INSTRUCTIONS

1) Place chipotle pepper, apricots and red pepper in a bowl; cover with water.

2) Let stand for 3 hours; drain and put into blender.

3) Add all other ingredients and blend on high speed, until well blended.

Asian Avocado Sauce

INGREDIENTS

1 ripe avocado

1 tsp red miso

6 tbsp cold water

1 tsp onion powder

1 tsp garlic powder

½ tsp cumin powder

½ tsp nama shoyu

1 tsp Himalayan sea salt

1 tbsp fresh lemon juice

½ cup Salba oil

PREPARATION INSTRUCTIONS

1) Add all ingredients to blender, except Salba oil, blending on high speed until smooth.

2) While still on high speed, slowly add oils to mixture. Blend until sauce is a creamy consistency.

Basil Walnut Pesto

INGREDIENTS

½ cup walnuts soaked
3 hours, drain and dry

1 clove garlic, minced

2 cups packed basil leaves

2 tbsp extra virgin olive oil

1 tsp sea salt

PREPARATION INSTRUCTIONS

1) Place all ingredients into a food processor or blender.

2) Process until well combined, but still chunky.

Creamy Chestnut Gravy

INGREDIENTS

1 cup soft chestnuts, clean-prepped*

½ cup dates, soaked for 1 hour, drained, cut in quarters

½ cup dark grapes, cut in half

1 cup warm water

½ tsp Bell's seasoning

½ tsp onion powder

~~ salt to taste

PREPARATION INSTRUCTIONS

1) Place all ingredients into food processor.

2) Blend until very fine and creamy.

3) Strain and store in glass jar in refrigerator.

NOTE:

*To clean-prep chestnuts, thoroughly wash and dry; remove any dark skins.

Dark Chocolate Fudge Sauce

INGREDIENTS

1 cup coconut milk

1 tbsp vanilla powder (or liquid)

¼ cup maple syrup

3 ounces raw cocoa powder

~~ touch sea salt

PREPARATION INSTRUCTIONS

1) Put all ingredients in blender and puree on high speed until mixture is completely smooth, stopping to scrape the sides as necessary.

Essence of Mango and Bell Pepper

INGREDIENTS

1 cup bell pepper diced

1 cup mango, peeled, diced

½ cup pineapple, diced

2 tbsp lemon juice

1 tsp nama shoyu

¼ cup almonds, soaked for 2 hours, washed

1 tbsp curry powder

¼ tsp garam masala

3 tbsp sesame oil

1 tbsp Salba oil

½ tsp turmeric powder

~~ raisins for garnish

PREPARATION INSTRUCTIONS

1) Put all ingredients – except raisins – into blender and puree on high speed until mixture is completely smooth, stopping to scrape the sides as necessary.

2) Garnish with raisins that have been rehydrated and plumped by soaking in water for about an hour.

Roasted Red Pepper Sauce

INGREDIENTS

3 red peppers

½ cup red palm oil

1 tbsp garlic powder

1 tbsp onion powder

~~ sea salt to taste

~~ cayenne

PREPARATION INSTRUCTIONS

1) Remove stems from peppers and cut into large dice.

2) Put in bowl and add 2 tbsp of the red palm oil, coat well and sprinkle lightly with salt. Place on Teflex sheet and dehydrate at 110° for approximately 6 hours, until peppers are pliable and soft.

3) Put peppers in blender, add garlic and onion powders, remainder of the red palm oil and salt to taste. Blend until completely liquefied.

4) Strain to remove pepper skin bits and pour red pepper liquid into a pan. Place pan on the bottom of the dehydrator and dehydrate at 110°.

5) Stirring every half hour, reduce liquid until it becomes the consistency of a sauce; it is ready when the sauce coats the back of a spoon.

Saffron Pine Nut Sauce

INGREDIENTS

½ cup raw pine nuts (soaked for 6 hours and drained

½ cup water

4 tbsp extra virgin olive oil

2 tbsp lemon juice

¼ tsp saffron powder (diluted in 1 tbsp warm water for 25 minutes)

3 drops nama shoyu

1 tsp maple syrup

~ salt to taste

PREPARATION INSTRUCTIONS

1) Combine all ingredients in blender at high speed until smooth (it will look like a sauce).

2) Mixture will thicken as it sits; to thin out, use more oil.

NOTE:

This sauce is great for a garnish.

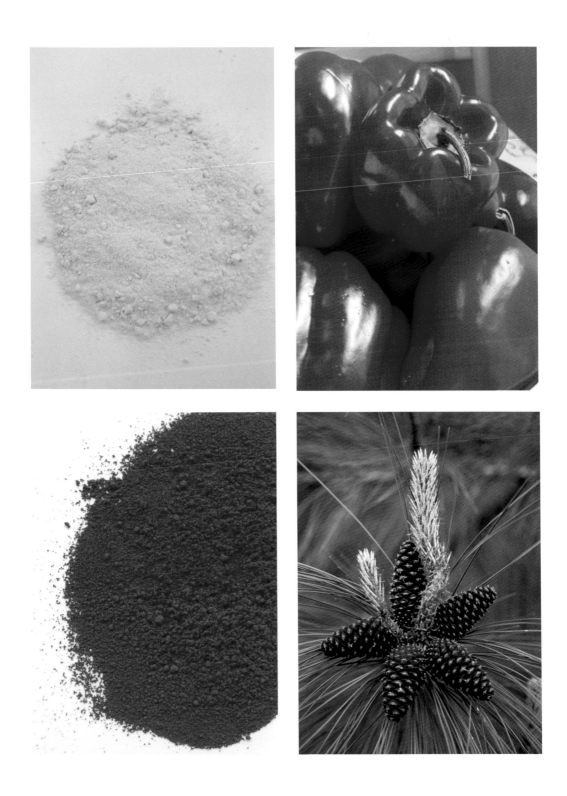

Spicy Mint Jelly Sauce

INGREDIENTS

1 cup coconut water

¼ cup fresh spearmint
leaves, diced

1 small jalapeño pepper,
seeded, diced

¼ cup Irish moss, soaked,
washed well, dried
(per package instructions)

2 tbsp white agave

1 tbsp lime juice

½ tsp garlic powder

1 tsp onion powder

½ tsp sea salt

PREPARATION INSTRUCTIONS

1) Place all ingredients into blender and
process on high speed until creamy.

2) Chill.

Wasabi Horseradish Sauce

INGREDIENTS

½ cup macadamia nuts

½ tbsp lemon juice

½ tsp sea salt

2 tbsp wasabi puree**

1 tbsp fresh horseradish root
(or prepared horseradish)

¼ cup cold water

⅛ cup extra virgin olive oil

PREPARATION INSTRUCTIONS

1) Soak macadamia nuts for 2 hours; dry.

2) Blend all ingredients except olive oil in
blender on high speed.

3) Scrape sides.

4) Finish by adding olive oil and blending
until smooth.

**Available in plastic tubes in Asian markets.

Wild Blueberry Ginger Sauce

INGREDIENTS

1 cup wild blueberries
2 tbsp agave
1 tbsp ginger juice
2 tbsp cold water
~~ 2 tbsp fresh lemon juice

PREPARATION INSTRUCTIONS

1) Place all ingredients into a blender and mix on high speed until smooth.

2) Strain and chill.

NOTE:

You may find you need more or less lemon juice, depending on the tartness of the blueberries.

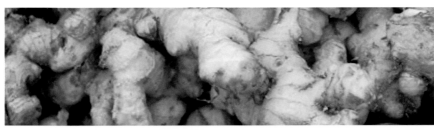

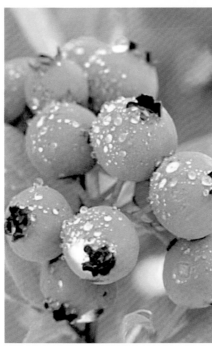

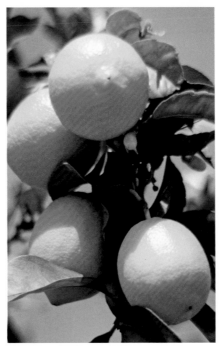

Soups

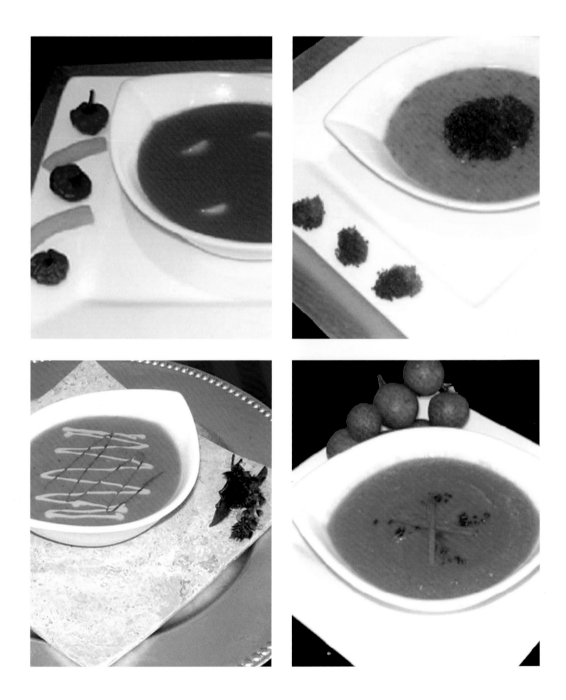

Avocado Crème with Chopped Vegetable Pastiche

INGREDIENTS

1 ½ large, ripe, avocados, peeled and cut into chunks

1 celery stalk, diced into large pieces

1 ½ tsp maple syrup

¼ cup spinach or arugula leaves

½ tsp sea salt

½ cup almond milk

½ cup coconut milk

½ tsp cayenne

1 large Gala apple, diced

1 ½ tsp nama shoyu

1 tsp fresh garlic, peeled and diced

VEGETABLE PASTICHE FOR GARNISH

very small diced red onions, red pepper, mango and cilantro, mixed

PREPARATION INSTRUCTIONS

1) Put all ingredients into blender, except the pastiche.

2) Blend until thoroughly mixed and to desired temperature.

3) Garnish top of avocado crème with spoonful of vegetable pastiche in middle of bowl.

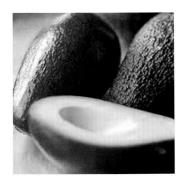
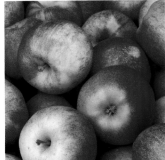
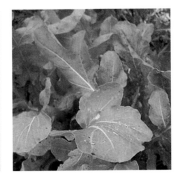

Beet Gazpacho

INGREDIENTS

1 pound fresh beets, peeled and chopped

½ red onion

1 small cucumber, peeled, seeds removed and diced

2 dates, pitted and soaked until soft

4 tbsp tahini

1 cup coconut water

¼ cup almond milk

½ cup carrot juice

1 tsp nama shoyu

~~ cayenne and sea salt to taste

1 cup mixed, small diced tart apple, red onion and peeled, seeded cucumber

PREPARATION INSTRUCTIONS

1) Place all ingredients – except final cup of mixed vegetables – in blender and process thoroughly.

2) Stir in the final cup of mixed vegetables.

3) Chill.

4) Serve garnished with small-diced apple.

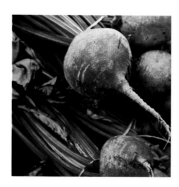
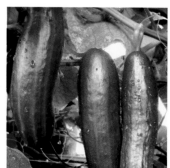
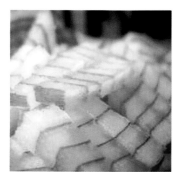

Bisque of Avocado

INGREDIENTS

3 large, ripe, avocados, peeled and cut into chunks

2 stalks green from celery, diced into large pieces

1 tbsp maple syrup

½ cup spinach or arugula leaves

1 tsp sea salt

1 cup almond milk

1 cup coconut milk

1 tsp cayenne

1 large Gala apple, diced

1 tbsp nama shoyu

1 tsp fresh garlic, peeled and diced

PREPARATION INSTRUCTIONS

1) Put almond milk and all other ingredients into blender.

2) Blend until thoroughly mixed and to desired temperature.

3) Serve with ginger pumpkin seeds.

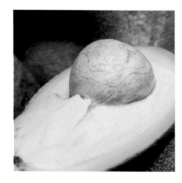
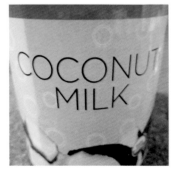
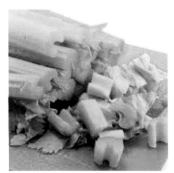

Butternut Squash and Ginger Soup with Spaghetti Squash Nest

INGREDIENTS

BUTTERNUT SQUASH AND GINGER SOUP

1 pound butternut squash, peeled, seeded and chopped for dehydrating

2 cups butternut squash, peeled, seeded and chopped for juicing

¼ cup butternut squash, peeled, seeded and chopped to be used raw

1½ cups water

2 tbsp chopped, peeled ginger

1 tbsp maple syrup

1 tbsp lemon juice

1 tbsp fresh chopped parsley, for garnish

SPAGHETTI SQUASH NEST

2 cups spaghetti squash, very ripe, shredded, peeled and soaked for 2 hours drained

1½ tbsp grape seed oil

1 tbsp apple cider vinegar

2 tbsp chopped scallion, green part only

salt and pepper to taste

PREPARATION INSTRUCTIONS

BUTTERNUT SQUASH AND GINGER SOUP

1) Arrange the 1 pound chopped butternut squash pieces on a Teflex sheet and dehydrate at 105° F for about 18 hours, or until dry.

2) Juice the 2 cups of the butternut squash. Discard the pulp; liquid should measure out to ½ cup juice.

3) Place the dried squash, water, squash juice, ginger, maple syrup, lemon juice and remaining ¼ cup of raw chopped squash into a blender and process until smooth. Pass the puree through a fine-mesh sieve; season to taste with salt and pepper.

SPAGHETTI SQUASH NEST

1) Using a fork, pull the drained shreds of squash into strands. Combine the squash, olive oil, vinegar and scallion in a bowl and toss to mix.

TO SERVE

1) Place spaghetti squash into the middle of a bowl, and cover with butternut squash soup. Garnish with fresh parsley.

Caribbean Chowder

INGREDIENTS

½ cup Brazil nuts, soaked for 2 hours

½ cup water

1 tbsp olive oil

1 tbsp fresh lemon juice

1 shallot

1 tsp nutritional yeast

1 tsp salt

¼ tsp chili powder

~~ black pepper

1 tbsp nama shoyu

GARNISH

1 cup chopped coconut meat

¼ cup diced red pepper

¼ cup minced celery

1 tbsp minced scallions

PREPARATION INSTRUCTIONS

1) Mix Brazil nuts and water in blender.

2) Strain through a fine strainer; discard pulp.

3) Blend nut milk and remaining ingredients in blender until completely smooth and creamy.

4) Season to taste.

5) Garnish with coconut meat, red pepper, celery and scallions.

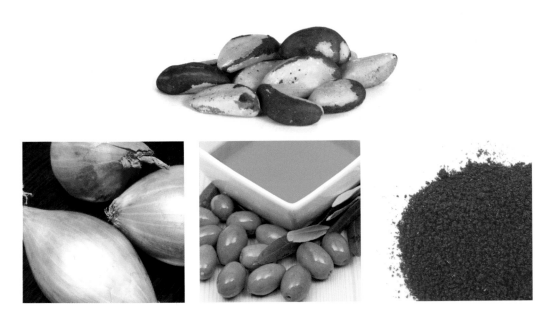

Carrot Ginger Soup

INGREDIENTS

6 extra large raw carrots, cut in chunks

1 tbsp white agave

1 tsp cinnamon

¼ tsp cayenne

3 cups almond milk

½ cup water

1 medium, ripe, avocado, pit removed, peeled and diced large

1 tsp minced fresh ginger

½ cup extra virgin olive oil

1 tbsp cilantro leaves

1 tbsp lime juice

PREPARATION INSTRUCTIONS

1) Wash carrots and remove stems and any sunburned (green) flesh.

2) Place almond milk, carrots, ginger, avocado, cinnamon, agave and cayenne in high-speed blender.

3) Blend for 30 seconds on high speed; slowly add the olive oil and water.

4) Serve with cilantro leaves. (To dilute consistency of soup, use more almond milk.)

Chilled Cantaloupe Ginger Bisque with Asian Longanberry Floaters

INGREDIENTS

2 cups ripe cantaloupe, peeled, large diced

½ cup carrots, peeled, large diced

¼ cup coconut water

~~ Hawaiian black lava sea salt

1 tsp ginger juice

1 tsp ground cinnamon powder

1 tbsp lime juice

2 to 3 longanberries per person, peeled, pitted, and cut in half

PREPARATION INSTRUCTIONS

1) Put all ingredients except longanberries and black sea salt into blender.

2) Blend on high speed until ingredients are mixed into a bisque consistency. Place in refrigerator to chill.

3) Place longanberries on bottom of bowl; pour very cold bisque over berries.

4) Sprinkle small amount of black lava sea salt on top just before serving.

Cream of Roasted Broccoli Bisque

INGREDIENTS

1 bunch broccoli florets, plus

1 tbsp additional florets

2 tbsp avocado, peeled and chopped

2 tsp onion, small diced

1 tsp garlic, peeled and small diced

⅓ cup parsley

2 cups almond milk

1 tbsp coconut butter

1 tsp nama shoyu

~~ Salba oil for coating

~~ sea salt to taste

~~ hemp hearts, for garnish

PREPARATION INSTRUCTIONS

1) Place all broccoli florets in bowl and flavor with Salba oil and sea salt. Dehydrate on Teflex sheet at 115° for 3½ hours.

2) Put all ingredients – except 1 tbsp broccoli florets and coconut butter – into blender and mix until soup becomes well blended.

3) Finish soup with coconut butter, by blending at high speed for a few last seconds.

4) Serve garnished with remaining broccoli florets and sprinkled with hemp hearts.

Creamy Consommé of Walnut and Dill

INGREDIENTS

4 cups water

1 cup grape seed oil

1 tbsp nama shoyu

1 clove fresh garlic

1 cup walnuts, soaked 8 hours and dried

1 tbsp ground cinnamon

1 tbsp fresh ginger

1 tbsp salt

1 tsp cayenne

1 tsp black pepper

2 tbsp fresh dill sprigs, chopped

PREPARATION INSTRUCTIONS

1) Pour liquid ingredients into blender first. Place remaining ingredients – except chopped dill – on top.

2) Blend on high speed, until mixture becomes a smooth soup.

3) Just prior to serving, stir chopped dill into soup. Garnish with a sprinkle of cinnamon walnut crumbles.

English Cucumber Soup with Carrot Salad and Tarragon Pine Nut Mayonnaise

INGREDIENTS

SOUP

2 English cucumbers, peeled and chopped

2½ tbsp fresh lemon juice

CARROT SALAD

2 large carrots, peeled, sliced on the extreme diagonal

1 tbsp thinly sliced scallions (white and green parts), sliced on the extreme diagonal

1 tbsp fresh lemon

1 tbsp cucumber, peeled and diced

1 tbsp olive oil

PINE NUT MAYONNAISE

½ cup raw pine nuts, soaked for 6 hours in water and drained

¼ cup water

3 tbsp grape seed oil

1 tsp lemon juice

2 tbsp chopped fresh tarragon leaves for garnish

~~ salt and pepper

PREPARATION INSTRUCTIONS

ENGLISH CUCUMBER SOUP

1) In high-speed blender, process cucumbers until smooth.

2) Add lemon juice, and flavor with salt and pepper; blend until warm. (If too thick, dilute with cold water.) Set Aside.

CARROT SALAD

1) In a bowl, combine carrots, scallion, cucumber, olive oil and lemon juice. Toss well to mix ingredients.

2) Season with salt and pepper. (Make this salad just before serving or keep it in the refrigerator.)

PINE NUT MAYONNAISE

1) In a high-speed blender, combine pine nuts, water, grape seed oil and lemon juice. Process until it has the consistency a mayonnaise.

2) Add tarragon leaves and season with salt and pepper. The mixture will thicken as it sits. If necessary, add more water. Put in a squeeze bottle and refrigerate.

TO SERVE

1) Place carrot salad in the center of each bowl. Ladle the soup around the salad. Squeeze pine nut mayonnaise in a ring around the salad, on top of the soup.

2) Top with chopped tarragon leaves across the soup and salad.

Hearty Green Vegetable Soup

INGREDIENTS

½ cup watercress

1 cup broccoli, diced

1 ½ cups kale leaves

1 cup spinach leaves

½ tbsp fresh peeled garlic

½ cup pineapple, diced

⅛ tsp chili powder

½ cup red onion, diced

2 ½ cups almond milk

½ cup coconut water

½ cup water

1 tbsp nama shoyu

salt and pepper to taste

2 tbsp red pepper, finely diced
(for garnish)

PREPARATION INSTRUCTIONS

1) Place all ingredients into blender (except diced red pepper) and blend at high speed; process until smooth. If mixture is too thick, dilute by adding water.

2) Flavor with salt and pepper. Garnish with 2 tbsp of finely diced red pepper.

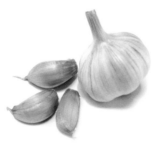

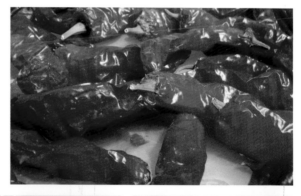

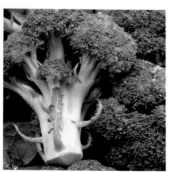

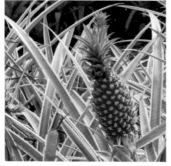

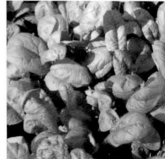

Horseradish Red Bell Pepper Soup with Mango Pillows and Lime Segments

INGREDIENTS

HORSERADISH RED BELL PEPPER SOUP

4 red bell peppers, juiced

1 tbsp horseradish juice

1 tbsp maple syrup

1 tbsp fresh lime juice

~~ salt and pepper to taste

MANGO PILLOWS

1 mango, peeled, pitted, chopped

2 tbsp Salba oil

1 tbsp Irish moss

1 tsp Himalayan sea salt

~~ fresh lime segments, for garnish

PREPARATION INSTRUCTIONS

HORSERADISH RED BELL PEPPER SOUP

1) Juice peppers in electric juicer; discard pulp.

2) Pour pepper juice into a bowl. Stir in horseradish juice, lime juice, maple syrup, salt and pepper. Place in refrigerator to chill.

MANGO PILLOWS

1) Combine all ingredients in blender; process until smooth.

2) Pour into a bowl; cover and refrigerate until slightly firm.

TO SERVE

1) Ladle chilled pepper soup into individual bowls. Garnish soup with small dollops of mango mixture and lime segments.

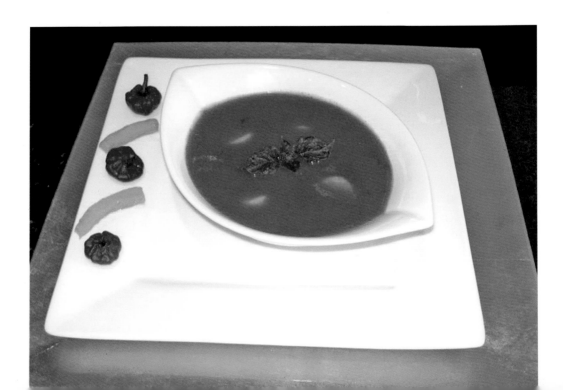

Miso Soup

INGREDIENTS

1 ½ cups water

2 tbsp nama shoyu

2 tbsp sesame oil

¼ cup white miso

1 ounce dried dulse, soaked in water for one half hour

~~ spiral zucchini and diced scallions, for garnish

PREPARATION INSTRUCTIONS

1) Squeeze excess water out of dulse between your hands.

2) Blend all ingredients in blender; serve warm.

3) Garnish top of soup with spiral zucchini and diced scallions.

Pineapple Cucumber Gazpacho

INGREDIENTS

3 ½ cups cucumber, chopped, peeled, diced

4 ½ cups chopped fresh pineapple, skin and core removed

½ cup of water

1 small jalapeño, seeded, diced

1 green onion, diced

3 tbsp extra virgin olive oil or macadamia oil

1 tbsp lemon juice

1 tbsp sea salt

4 tbsp cilantro leaves

2 tbsp raw macadamia nuts, finely chopped, for garnish

PREPARATION INSTRUCTIONS

1) Place 3 ½ cups pineapple, 2 tbsp cilantro leaves, and remaining ingredients (except macadamia nuts) and blend thoroughly.

2) Add the remaining cup of chopped pineapple to gazpacho; stir well.

3) Pour into bowls, garnish top with remaining cilantro leaves and macadamia nuts.

Pumpkin Patch Potage

INGREDIENTS

1 ½ cups pumpkin, pared, diced

½ cup avocado

1 cup water

1 cup almond milk

1 tbsp agave

1 tbsp coconut butter

1 tsp fresh ginger, grated

½ tsp cinnamon powder

½ tsp fresh lemon juice

¼ tsp sea salt

PREPARATION INSTRUCTIONS

1) Flavor pumpkin pieces with small amount of grape seed oil and salt.

2) Place on Teflex sheet and dehydrate at 105° for 3 hours.

3) Put all ingredients, including pumpkin, into blender and blend on high speed until well blended.

4) Strain; store in refrigerator in glass jar.

NOTE:

Serve with crispy pear chip on top, sprinkled with black pepper.

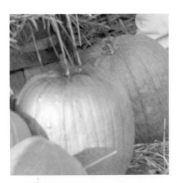
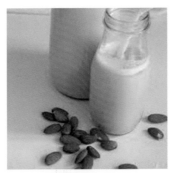
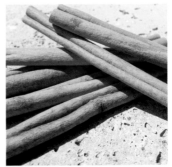

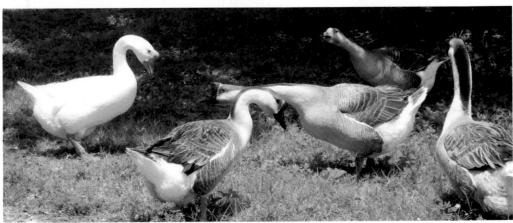

Roasted Golden Cauliflower Potage with Wilted Lettuce and Caramelized Onions

INGREDIENTS

CAULIFLOWER POTAGE

1 small head yellow cauliflower

2 cloves garlic, peeled; large diced

½ Vidalia onion, large diced

3 cups almond milk

~ sea salt to taste

~ cayenne to taste

WILTED LETTUCE

1 cup lettuce, well washed and dried

2 tsp grape seed oil

~ sea salt to taste

CARAMELIZED ONIONS

1 red onion, peeled, sliced small

2 tbsp apple cider vinegar

1 tbsp maple syrup

½ tsp sea salt

PREPARATION INSTRUCTIONS

1) Cut cauliflower into florets and wash well in mixture of water and dash of peroxide. Let soak for 15 minutes in mixture; drain and dry.

2) Place in bowl and flavor with sea salt; coat with oil. Add garlic and Vidalia onion.

3) Place on Teflex sheet in dehydrator on 115° for 6 hours. Remove; put into blender with almond milk, salt and cayenne. Blend well; set aside.

4) Peel red onion; cut into small slices. Place into bowl with apple cider vinegar, sea salt, and maple syrup. Marinate for 3 hours. Drain and dehydrate on Teflex sheet at 115° until tender.

5) Wash and dry lettuce well and cut into julienne strips. Flavor with grape seed oil and sea salt; dehydrate on Teflex sheet at 115° for about 20 minutes.

6) Pour cauliflower soup into individual bowls; garnish with wilted lettuce and caramelized onions.

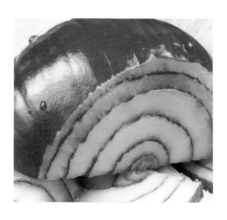

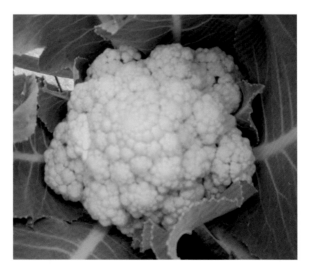

Spring Garden Fennel Asparagus Soup with Caramelized Fennel Shavings

INGREDIENTS

3 cups asparagus

½ cup fennel, diced

1 large ripe avocado

2 celery stalks

¼ cup spinach leaves

1 tbsp lemon juice

1 cup Granny Smith apple, diced with skin

1 tsp garlic powder

1 cup water

1 tsp ground nutmeg

1 tbsp nama shoyu

~~ sea salt to taste

~~ shaved caramelized fennel and pieces of roasted asparagus for garnish

PREPARATION INSTRUCTIONS

1) Wash asparagus; remove hard white parts; cut into very large dice.

2) Wash and remove white bottoms from celery stalks; cut into large dice.

3) Wash and cut fennel into large dice.

4) Core apple, leaving skin on and cut into large dice.

5) Wash spinach leaves.

6) Place asparagus, celery, fennel, apple and spinach into juice. Juice all to make a vegetable stock.

7) Put vegetable stock into blender; add all other ingredients. Process until mixture is well blended.

8) Serve garnished with caramelized fennel shavings and pieces of roasted asparagus.

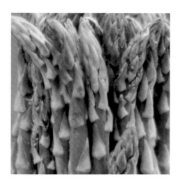 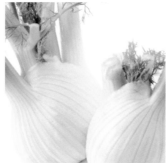 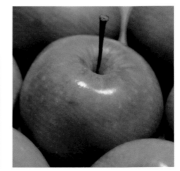

Sunrise Borscht

INGREDIENTS

¼ pound fresh beets, peeled
and chopped

1 cup coconut water

¼ cup almond milk

½ cup carrot juice

1 tsp nama shoyu

2 dates, pitted and soaked

1 tbsp tahini

~~cayenne and sea salt
to taste

¼ cucumber, peeled, seeds
removed and diced, for garnish

1 tbsp fresh dill, for garnish

PREPARATION INSTRUCTIONS

1) Place coconut water, almond milk and beets into blender. Process thoroughly.

2) Add all remaining ingredients except chopped cucumber and dill; blend until creamy.

3) Chill.

4) Serve garnished with small-diced cucumber and sprig of dill.

Swiss Chard Fantasy Soup

INGREDIENTS

2 cups coconut milk

1 tsp garlic powder

1 tsp onion powder

½ cup olive oil

6 ounces Swiss chard, washed
well and dried

1 tsp ground clove

1 tsp Himalayan sea salt

8 ounces green grapes, frozen

1 tsp nama shoyu

4 ounces spinach

PREPARATION INSTRUCTIONS

1) Place all ingredients except oil into blender. Blend at high speed.

2) When mixture is creamy, slowly add in the oil.

3) Drizzle with saffron pine nut sauce.

NOTE:

This dish can be served warm or cold.

Tropical Papaya Pineapple Soup

INGREDIENTS

¼ ripe pineapple, cut into
large chunks

1 ripe papaya, seeds removed,
cut into large chunks

4 oz fresh mint leaves

1 tbsp agave

8 oz coconut water

juice of 1 fresh lime

1 tsp fresh peeled ginger

~~ lime zest, for garnish

~~ pineapple chunks,
for garnish

~~ papaya chunks, for garnish

PREPARATION INSTRUCTIONS

1) Put all ingredients in blender; mix on high speed until well blended.

2) Place in refrigerator and cool until desired temperature.

3) Serve with small chunks of pineapple or papaya (or both) and fresh grated lime zest.

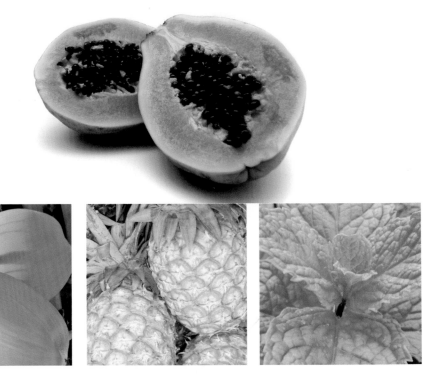

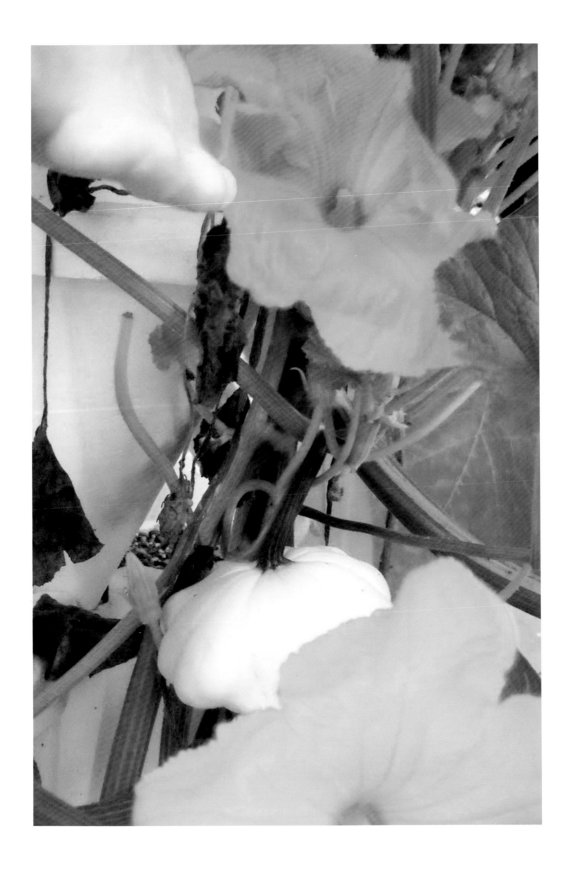

Meal Menu Suggestions

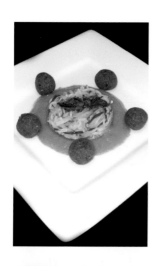
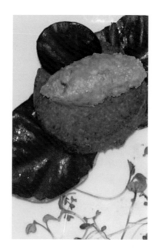
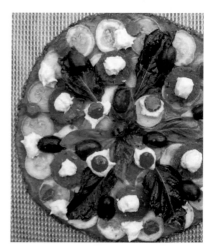
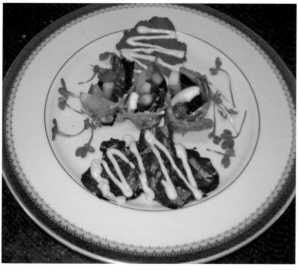
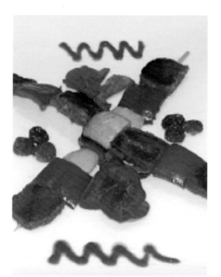

Amazing Veggie Burger

Arugula Fennel, Apple,
Pomegranate Salad

Amazing Veggie Burger
Avocado Dressing

Apple Ginger Citrus Delights

Curry Spring Salad

Swiss Chard Fantasy Soup
Saffron Pine Nut Sauce

Curry Spring Salad
Mint Citrus Almond Chutney
Spicy Pecans

Kiwi Banana Chia Vanilla Pudding

Hemp Hearts Spring Salad

Tropical Papaya Pineapple Soup

Hemp Hearts Spring Salad
Spinach and Nasturtium Leaves
Grapefruit Segments, Avocado

Coconut Macaroons

Kelp Noodle Swirl

Salad of Arugula, Micro Greens
Grapefruit Segments and Watermelon

Kelp Noodle Swirl
Asian Ginger Emulsion
Edamame, Brunoise of Red Pepper

Fudgy Chocolate Torte

Lamb Chop, Spicy Mint Jelly Sauce

Beet Gazpacho

Lamb Chop
Spicy Mint Jelly Sauce

Roasted Lima Beans and Pearl Onions

Key Lime Torte
Wild Blueberry Ginger Sauce

Moroccan Sun Kebabs

Chilled Cantaloupe Ginger Bisque

Moroccan Sun Kebabs

Apricot Barbecue Sauce

Tropical Pineapple Salsa

Key Lime Torte

Pad Thai Pasta of Zucchini

Carrot Ginger Soup

Pad Thai Pasta of Zucchini

Chilled Berries Chia Mousse

Pasta Primo "Bella Serra"

Creamy Consommé of Walnut and Dill

Pasta Primo "Bella Serra"

Vanilla Gogi Berry Pudding

Pattypan Angel Hair
with Heaven Drops

Cream of Roasted Broccoli Bisque

Pattypan Angel Hair with Heaven Drops
Roasted Red Pepper Sauce

Almond Pomegranate Tapioca

"Rawsage" Pizza

Krunchy, Krispy Kale Kracklin's

"Rawsage" Pizza

Petite Salad of Arugula
Sweet & Sour Red Onions
Herb Vinaigrette

Caramelized Peach Torte

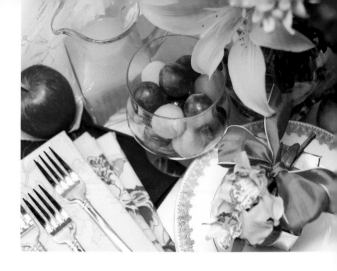

Savory Crepe Roll-up

Horseradish Red Bell Pepper Soup

Savory Crepe Roll-up
Selection of Vegetables
Wasabi Horseradish Sauce

Cinnamon Banana Ice Cream
Banana Slices and Chocolate Chips

Sea and Land Asian Salad

Sunrise Borscht

Sea and Land Asian Salad
Sweet Miso Dressing

Double Dark Chocolate Pudding
Sesame Brittle Crunch
Fresh Garden Strawberries

Spaghetti of Zucchini, Pesto Emulsion

Roasted Golden Cauliflower Potage

Spaghetti of Zucchini

Nutty Pesto Emulsion

Vanilla Peach and Mixed Berry Dreams
Macadamia Nut Clouds

Stuffed Roasted Red Peppers

Miso Soup

Stuffed Roasted Red Peppers
Cilantro Curry Hummus
Ponzu Ginger Dipping Sauce

Macadamia-Mango Delight
Coulis of Wild Blueberry

Turkey Leggings, Creamy Chestnut Gravy

Pumpkin Patch Soup
Turkey Leggings
Creamy Chestnut Gravy

Granny Smith's Apple Stuffing

Root Vegetable Pine Nut Whip

Chunky Cherry Grapefruit Relish

Pumpkin Mousse
Candied Pecans

Young Coconut Pad Thai

Pineapple Cucumber
Gazpacho Soup

Young Coconut Pad Thai

Chia Mango Mint Mousse

Zucchini Fettuccine Alfredo

Creamy Consommé of Walnut and Dill

Zucchini Fettuccini Alfredo

Wake-Me Shake-Me Chocolate Coffee
Mousse
Almond Brittle Crunch

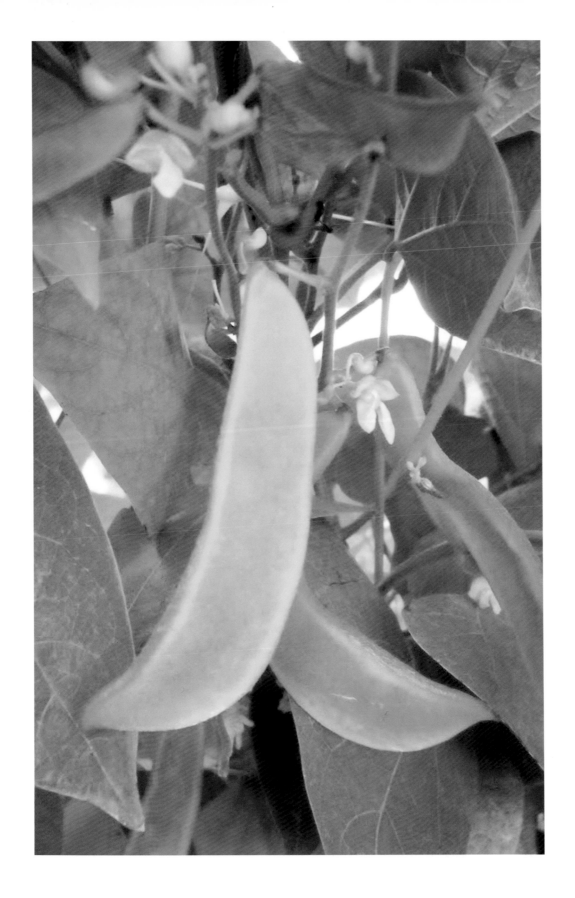

Index

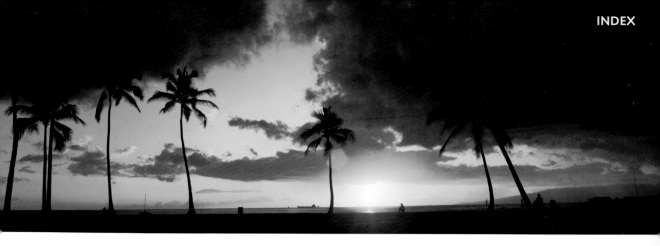

Chef Salomon Montezinos
Owner/Operator/Chef
Restaurants

Restaurant Déjà Vu
Philadelphia, Pennsylvania

Montezinos Restaurant
Palm Beach, Florida

Montezinos Restaurant
Orlando, Florida

Restaurant Angelique
Boca Raton, Florida

Restaurant Awards
A Sampling

Déjà-Vu Restaurant – USA's Top French Restaurant, USA Today; What's Hot for 1987 and 1988, Food and Wine Magazine; Ambassador Award; Grand Award of Excellence, The Wine Spectator; One of the Most Creative Chefs in America, MD Magazine; Cartier Award; The Best Wine List Around, Philadelphia Magazine; Most Romantic Restaurant in the USA, Food and Wine; Craig Claiborne's Golden Spoon Award; Excellence in Dining, Main Liner/United Airlines Magazine; Top of the Table Competition Award, Hospitality Magazine.

Montezinos Restaurants – Palm Beach, Florida and Orlando, Florida - Rated one of the hottest new restaurants in America by Esquire Magazine; Rated Best Chef of 1990 by Orlando Lifestyle Magazine; Rated Best Chef in Central Florida by Florida Magazine; Named one of Florida's people to watch in 1990 – Sal Montezinos, Culinary Master – by Orlando Magazine; November 1989 proclaimed "Montezinos Month" by Mayor Fredericks of Orlando; Received Key to the City of Orlando. Rated Four Stars, Palm Beach Post and Miami Herald.

Angelique Restaurant – Rated one of the best restaurants in America by Esquire Magazine; Rated Four Stars by the Palm Beach Post.

A Taste of Restaurant Testimonials

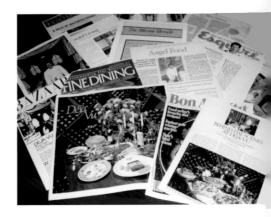

"Referring to Montezinos simply as a chef, even a master chef, is like saying Mozart was just a guy who wrote music." *−XS Magazine*

"Montezinos' cooking style is 'cuisine libre'. It is inventive; in short, it is his own." *−Travel/Holiday Magazine*

"Montezinos' Swiss schooling intensified his dedication to health and nutrition, and its influence is evident in every phase of his cooking." *−Harper's Bazaar*

"One of the hottest new restaurants in America. Montezinos was one of the first in this country to combine Eastern and Western flavors, and he is a master of the genre." *−Esquire Magazine*

"His way with seasoning is unique in the Palm Beaches and can only be described as wizardry." *−Weekly Business/Ft. Lauderdale News/Sun-Sentinel*

"One of the most creative chefs in the United States today." *−Food & Wine Magazine*

"Montezinos' cooking is fascinating for its melding of seasonings and spices… food of the highest caliber with the best balanced nutrition." *−MD Magazine*

"When Sal Montezinos closed Déjà vu, his highly acclaimed Philadelphia restaurant, the uproar could be heard up and down the East Coast…Sal is the quintessential owner/chef." *−Florida Home & Garden*

"Salomon Montezinos orchestrates the dinners to be almost magically memorable."
–*Chocolatier Magazine*

"Four stars for personal style and genius for rich and brilliant seasoning seldom found in today's restaurant kitchens. Sal Montezinos is a chef of the new order." –*Miami Herald*

"Salomon Montezinos has made area gastronomes see culinary stars." –*Palm Beach Post*

"Sal is not only tireless, but impassioned about his work."
–Nationally published food critic John Mariani
(Esquire Magazine, Fine Dining Magazine, USA Today)

"Montezinos is a perfectionist and a visionary, with the energy and imagination of a dozen royal chefs." –*Bon Appétit Magazine*

"Sal Montezinos has world travel experience and more gastronomic ideas than he knows what to do with." –*Chicago Tribune*

"Salomon Montezinos turns out French dishes of extraordinary quality." –*Gourmet Magazine*

"One of the most outstanding lunches I've ever had." –Mrs. George (Barbara) Bush

"Unlike anything you've experienced before except in a dream." –*Fine Dining Magazine*

"Only an artist like Montezinos could conduct the astounding variety of flavors into a harmonious symphony of tastes." –*Goodlife Magazine*

"Salomon Montezinos has a hard act to follow – himself." –*Orlando Magazine*

"The finest restaurant in the world." –Director-Gastronome Francis Ford Coppola

"No one in the South is doing better seafood than Montezinos." –*Esquire Magazine*

"You are a blooming genius, sir." –Zack Hanle, New York Editor, *Bon Appétit Magazine*

Chef Sal's Class Attendees Sampling of Testimonials

"Chef Sal has an encyclopedic knowledge of food development from his 55 years of experience as a internationally renowned chef. He presents and demonstrates this knowledge to his students in a very easy to understand format during his classes, and offers the results of his expertise with food for his students to enjoy. " *—Class Attendee*

"While nearly all chefs have a large, rotund physique, Chef Sal's physique is trim and athletic, bearing testimony to the fact that he practices what he preaches and it has paid off handsomely in his health." *—Class Attendee*

"Since applying Chef Sal's food secrets in my kitchen, my own health and outlook on life has dramatically improved." *—Class Attendee*

"I've gone to tons of vegan classes and tasted lots of raw vegan food, but never have I been to a class as professional and perfectly educational like what Chef Sal puts forth. The most educational and wonderful food EVER! " *—Class Attendee*

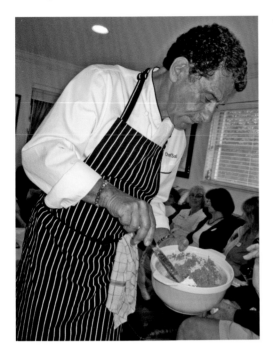

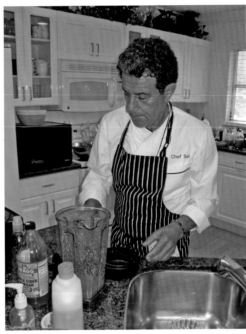

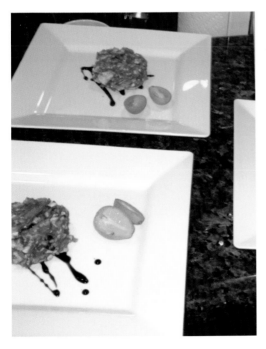

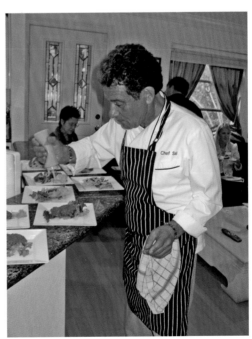

March 1, 2011

Dear Chef Montezinos:

If you were to ask anyone who knows me what my favorite meal is, without hesitation, they would say "He's a steak and loaded baked potato guy". Now, at 47, and after having meat and potatoes 3 or 4 times a week for years and years, for me to have transitioned so easily to a meat-free diet is nothing short of miraculous. I have never felt, or looked healthier!

I don't think you could know what an impact your extensive culinary knowledge, your encouragement and guidance in cooking class has been to me, and I wanted to thank you from the bottom of my heart!

I never would have thought that a raw vegan diet would be something I would have been the least bit interested in–- but the manner in which you prepare meals– the flavors, the presentation, and the ease with which you prepare full menus has made me a believer, and one of your biggest fans! I am thoroughly enjoying this new diet.

Actually, I hesitate to use the word "diet" in this letter, because I realize this is much more than a temporary eating plan, **you have shown me that being vegan is a lifestyle**, not simply a phase!

All of my praise isn't simply a feeling I have either, I have actually had a live blood analysis done recently, and my blood tests were much improved! So I know this is the best lifestyle for me, and I look forward to learning more recipes, with the wonderful recipes in your cookbook, and have already converted of my carnivore friends to join me in my healthy lifestyle path!

Thank you again Chef, you are an artist, a mentor, and I sincerely appreciate ALL you have done for me.

Sincerely,

Darrell Hart

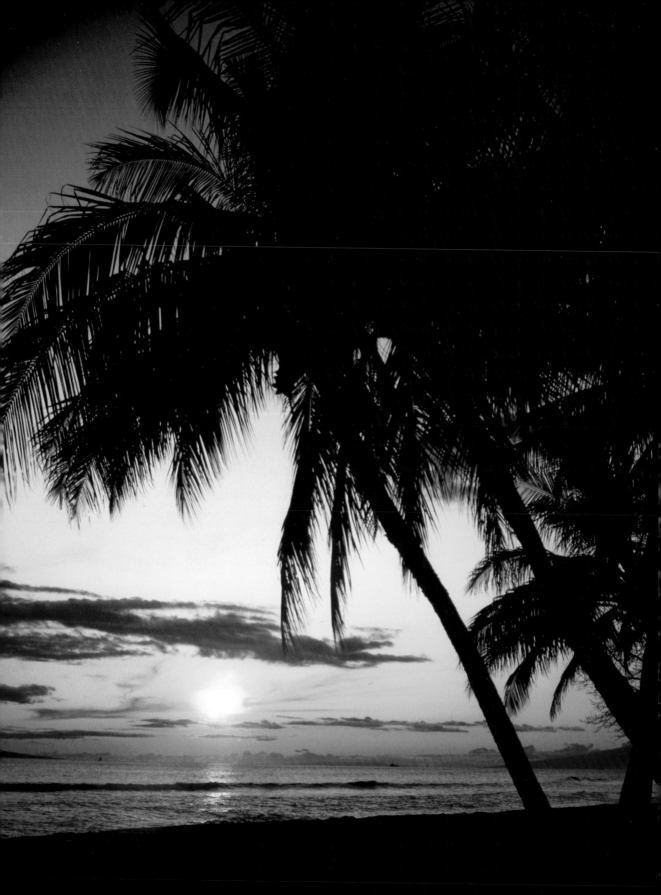

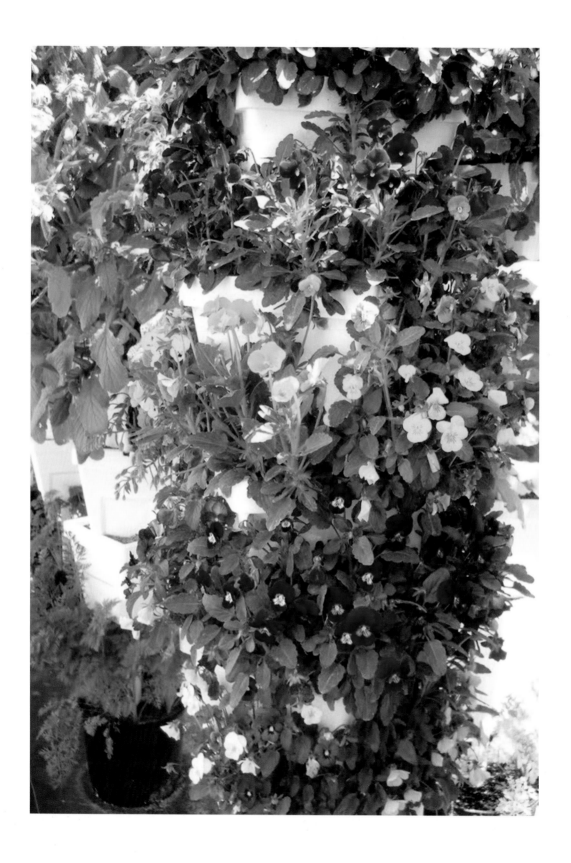